SOUND
MEDICINE

How to Use the Ancient Science of
Sound to Heal the Body and Mind

KULREET CHAUDHARY, MD

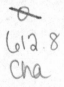

HARPER WAVE

An Imprint of HarperCollinsPublishers

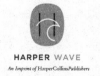

SOUND MEDICINE. Copyright © 2020 by Kulreet Chaudhary. All rights reserved. Printed in the United States of America. No part of this book may be used or reproduced in any manner whatsoever without written permission except in the case of brief quotations embodied in critical articles and reviews. For information, address HarperCollins Publishers, 195 Broadway, New York, NY 10007.

HarperCollins books may be purchased for educational, business, or sales promotional use. For information, please email the Special Markets Department at SPsales@harpercollins.com.

FIRST EDITION

Designed by Bonni Leon-Berman

Library of Congress Cataloging-in-Publication Data has been applied for.

ISBN 978-0-06-286733-9

20 21 22 23 24   LSC   10 9 8 7 6 5 4 3 2 1

This book is dedicated to Sri Sakthi Amma,
my guru and the inspiration for this project.
Throughout the writing of this book, Amma
not only gave me a deeper understanding and
appreciation for the brilliance of the Siddha tradition
but she also profoundly opened my heart and mind
to the science of mantras. I will be eternally grateful
for this priceless gift.

Om Namo Narayani.

CONTENTS

INTRODUCTION

This is a story of discovery and rediscovery—in my own life and in history. In my personal story, there was the uncovering by my mother of her own lost past, the traditions of her native India—which occurred in her midlife, ironically, when she moved to America. By chance her Western doctor suggested, after she complained of feeling run down, that she see a meditation teacher who could help her to start a Transcendental Meditation (TM) practice. This began, for my mother, an incredible journey deep into the ancient tradition of mantra meditation and Ayurvedic medicine in Indian culture, even as she continued to live out the American dream in Southern California.

It was my mother's discovery that led to my own profound rediscovery. Having started my own mantra practice at age nine alongside my mother, I carried our familial immersion in ancient Indian medicine forward into my professional life, transforming my neurology practice into an integrative medicine clinic and, ultimately, moving my own family *back* to India, where I now live and work as an Ayurvedic physician. Just as my paternal grandfather was a village doctor in Gujjarwal, India, I now also work as a physician in a small rural town outside of Vellore, India. I feel, however, more like a global village doctor: People travel from all over the world for consultations and treatments with me and other doctors at the Ayurvedic and Siddha medicine center in Tamil Nadu's local hospital that was created by Amma, my spiritual teacher.

From a historic vantage, the narrative of discovery and rediscovery, though broader in scope, is similar to my own. Approximately eight thousand years ago, Siddha medicine—an extremely potent form of medicine, largely shrouded in mystery—was practiced by Indian sages in South India. These spiritual masters developed many of the mantras we know today, the sounds connecting them to a reservoir of divine energy and forming the cornerstone of their practice. Around three thousand years later, Ayurvedic medicine took root in North India, sharing some of the same concepts as Siddha medicine, including an adapted mantra practice, in addressing diet, exercise, and lifestyle. In Sanskrit, *ayur* means "life" and *veda* means "knowledge," and this medical system conveyed not only the wisdom of life but also how to enact it, with notable results, in a daily way.

Yet over the course of history—beginning in 1858, when the British Raj began its century-long rule in India—these ancient spiritual and medical lineages have slowly vanished. Along with their system of governance, the British brought a permeating sense of superiority, and soon many of these sophisticated and effective Indian medical traditions gave way to more modern views, particularly those of Western medicine.

More recently, however, the tenets of these ancient systems have reemerged, under the guise of new theories and research. Beginning with the advent of quantum physics in the early 1900s, and just fifty years later moving through the invention of the ultrasound in Western medicine, which showed that sound waves could capture images of internal organs, and onward to the 1990s, with the emergence of biofield science—the powerful impact of sound medicine on the body has begun to be recognized once again.

It is here that my story and history converge. When I moved to Tamil Nadu two years ago, it was to help establish the Ayurvedic and Siddha medicine center, yes, but also to work with Amma, who is, in the traditional sense of the term, my spiritual guru. As it was done in ancient times, when would-be physicians received the wisdom of tradition as a rigorous experiential process, she is teaching me the art and practice of Siddha medicine. Amma was born in Vellore and raised as a boy in a loving family with little means until, at the age of sixteen, while riding on a bus he felt a beam of energy shoot through him and project upward into the sky. The Goddess Narayani, the divine mother, appeared in the image projected in the sky. This was understood to be the proclamation that she was returning to earth with Amma as her avatar. An avatar, as the guru and author of the classic book *Autobiography of a Yogi*, Paramahansa Yogananda, once said, "is born not to show us how great he was, but to give us hope that the state of consciousness he had attained, we too can attain." Though the concept of avatars is widely accepted in Indian culture, I realize it is an unfamiliar, and perhaps inconceivable, notion for Westerners. To help put it into context, Buddha was considered to be an avatar of the Hindu God Vishnu. (All avatars, however, are not founders of major religions or well-known leaders—some carry on their spiritual mission outside of the spotlight.)

Since Narayani's image appeared and Amma was claimed as a divine being, she (the pronoun now used to describe Amma given the presence of Narayani within) has created a spiritual compound containing several different temples, implemented educational programs and environmental initiatives throughout India, and is visited for spiritual guidance by the presidents of India as well as spiritual and political leaders from all over the world.

Amma also happens to be in possession of some of the most closely guarded texts of Siddha medicine. These are the palm leaf manuscripts, written in ancient dialect on dried palm leaves, cut into the shape of rectangles. Over the centuries, as the leaves decayed, duplicates have been copied onto new sets of dried palm leaves, but their wisdom dates back eight thousand years. These texts, in addition to being a treasure trove of historical and ethnographic information about the Siddhas, also include an elaborate description of their traditional medical system, including herbal formulations and the original mantras used for both healing and spiritual enlightenment.

Through Amma, I am learning about the enigmatic and impressive Siddhas—described in the Upanishads, a text that is part of the oldest existing Sanskrit literature in India, as possessed of "superhuman powers." The Siddhas were spiritual sages, expansively perceptive and highly attuned to nature—they even created mantra practices to mimic, as well as resonate with, the sounds of the natural world. We have learned from oral history, and the palm leaf manuscripts indicate, that this system of medicine is inextricably linked to a spiritual view of the universe. Their understanding of well-being encompassed both physical health and mental balance—one cannot be achieved without the other. Their physiological understanding of the body and health is predicated on a strong connection to a massless energy—what they called Brahman. The Siddhas put themselves through rigorous trials to reach a place of both enlightenment and optimum health—fasting, taking vows of silence, creating and ingesting complex herbal formulations, engaging in lengthy mantra practices. In so doing, they achieved a spiritual existence concomitant with excellent physical health and endurance.

When Ayurvedic medicine emerged, three thousand years later, it adapted some of the same medical concepts—such as viewing biological energies as distinct dosha types—as well as the Siddha mantra practice. Though both systems encourage a spiritual practice for its physiological benefits, Siddha medicine tends to be austere and all-encompassing, whereas Ayurvedic medicine is more accessible to everyone. Still, Ayurveda is a natural approach to health built on ancient scientific methods, such as the use of sound and vibrational medicine and diet and herbal formulas, to balance the body and mind.

Both systems offer, as Western medicine has slowly and methodically begun to glean, an early glimpse into the potent use of sound and vibration to alter human biology, capable of healing both body and mind. There have been times when I feel as if I am living backward, or watching a history reel rewind, when I read of new revelations about sound medicine or discuss an intriguing new medical field with colleagues—such as epigenetics—that seem, to me, to be a revival of Siddha and Ayurvedic principles.

This confluence between Eastern and Western medicine is what has compelled me over the last two years to stay strong in the face of so many challenges, both logistical and personal, in this rural Indian village—this idea that I am both looking back into a hidden past while also finding myself at the front lines of modern medicine. We have come an incredible distance in terms of understanding sound medicine, but as I chronicle in this book, I believe there is an undiscovered landscape of sound healing that we have yet to fully traverse.

SOUND MEDICINE

1

MY MANTRA

We are slowed down sound and light waves, a walking bundle of
frequencies tuned to the cosmos.

—ALBERT EINSTEIN

Until I was four years old, I lived in Punjab, India, with
my parents, my younger sister, my grandparents, and my
great-grandparents all piled into one house, each generation
looking after the next. Our green, three-story house was built
by my great-grandfather and surrounded by acres of farmland;
there were buffalo that lived in a little section of their own
just beyond the back door with goats and chickens roaming
beyond. Practically speaking, we were lucky because we had
the means to live comfortably in India. Emotionally speaking, life felt charmed because our home was bursting with
love. The door was unlocked in the morning and left open all
day for neighbors and friends and family to come and go as
they pleased. There was always something simmering in the
kitchen, giving way to the most amazing smells—everything

we ate was cooked from scratch, right down to the home-churned butter, and much of our food was harvested from the land surrounding our house. Our home was always filled with conversation, about daily matters such as what was happening with the farm but also searching ones, as we considered how to best care for our community or make the right choices in life.

Like most people in Punjab, we practiced Sikhism, a religion that originated in the region in the fifteenth century. Sikhs believe in one Supreme Being and practice compassion, honesty, and selfless service. The religion also encourages meditation as a means to feel God's presence.

And yet, although my family went to the gurdwara, the Sikh temple, every Sunday and followed the basic tenets of the religion, we did not meditate. This was not unusual: Most Indians stopped meditating nearly a hundred years ago. In the decades following the installation of the British government in 1858, beginning their century-long rule, the spiritual lineage of India was disrupted. Many of the ancient practices, such as meditation, North India's five-thousand-year-old Ayurvedic medical system, and the eight-thousand-year-old Siddha medicine tradition that had emerged in the south, slowly unraveled. The Brits considered their own systems to be superior and, over time, their governance eroded the ancient Indian customs and the faith with which they were practiced. The British even went so far as to destroy some of the ancient Indian spiritual records, literally obliterating the wisdom of the ages. Soon, Western medicine—with its focus on anatomy—had replaced the established holistic model combining body, mind, and spirit. An inferiority complex took hold in India and we began to look yearningly west, believing that there was something better in America, something perhaps even more prosperous and exceptional. It was a broad and shapeless promise—and all the more powerful for it. This yearning became a movement, and eventually it was simply what striving upper-middle-class Indian families did: They moved to America.

My parents were no exception. In 1977, they left the comfort and steadiness of our life in Punjab and set up a new home for just the four of us in Southern California. Within a year, they both had steady, well-paying jobs—my father as an engineer, my mother as a physical therapist (both occupations they'd had in India). Within five years, we were living in a five-bedroom house in Riverside County, my parents each drove their own Mercedes, and my sister and I were thriving at school. In short, my parents had achieved the American dream.

And they were totally stressed out.

Not long after they'd moved to the United States and achieved their goals (the house, the cars, a stellar education for their children), my mother got profoundly sick for the first time in her life. She was run down; her weight dropped suddenly, she experienced heart palpitations, and she felt a general sense of anxiety. Her physician referred her to an endocrinologist, who told her she'd developed a thyroid condition. After prescribing medication for the palpitations she was experiencing as a result of her thyroid condition, he surprised my mother by recommending that she begin practicing Transcendental Meditation. He was not a doctor of integrative medicine, a practice that was just starting to gain a foothold in the United States at that time, so it was a matter of chance, or perhaps fate, that this American doctor would hand her the name of

a meditation teacher, thus beginning my mother's journey—
and subsequently my own—into the ancient traditions of our
native culture.

Within six months, my mother's thyroid had normalized,
the bold sparkle was back in her eye, and she was convinced
that silently chanting a mantra had played a significant role in
her recovery. She was so convinced, in fact, that she brought my
sister and me to see her teacher, too. We were only seven and
nine years old, respectively, at the time. I'll never forget the details of that day: Sitting in a home filled with lush, green plants
with a strong smell of incense filling the room, my mother introduced us to Norma, a dark-haired woman with warm eyes
and a constant smile.

When Norma leaned over to whisper my bija mantra into my
ear, it sounded like beautiful nonsense, a sound without meaning. I felt certain Norma was offering some kind of enchant-
ment. Which is, in a way, what the bija mantra can feel like. *Bija*
means "seed" in Sanskrit, and in the Vedic tradition, one of the
oldest recorded spiritual practices in India, this mantra prompts
growth and transformation. This "seed mantra" was created to
encompass sounds that cannot be translated into literal meaning
but that utilize the power of tonal vibration to create balance and
peace in the body and mind. Many of us, in fact, have already
chanted a bija mantra at some point in our lives: The *Om* intoned at the beginning and end of yoga classes is a classic example. More broadly, the Vedic disciples believed that bija mantras
intimately connect a person to the energy field we call universal
consciousness that runs through—and connects—all matter in
the universe. Sound medicine, particularly as practiced by the

ancients, uses the tones of nature—which vibrate at a specific frequency—to help restore balance within us, and also to forge a connection with this larger energy field.

I have chanted this mantra nearly every day since Norma offered it to me thirty-six years ago, and it has profoundly altered my life in ways that I could not have anticipated. Initially, my bija mantra gave me access to a protected place that I would not have ever found otherwise. For a child to sit in complete silence for ten minutes twice a day—the amount of time, initially, that I silently chanted this mantra—is a challenging endeavor. But in learning to do so, I became aware of an inner reality I had not discovered before. At only nine years old, I found there was a place within me that was also outside of me—which was my childlike way of understanding my connection to the life force. Over time, this place became a centering retreat. I came to understand that I was something more than what I saw or felt or perceived in the world around me. And *whatever* that something more was, it was profoundly quiet and calming. My bija mantra was the key to a space inside of me that was always peaceful, independent of anything that was happening in my life. Once I learned that this existed, the physical world could no longer dominate me.

As my mother's commitment to ancient Indian tradition grew, she began to explore possible explanations for the mystical world that was unfolding before her. She had come to profoundly believe in a universal consciousness, and the notion that there is a sea of energy that connects us. She had also come to accept, as Vedic tradition proposes, that our individual spiritual efforts can create consequential change not only in ourselves but also in the world. As part of her exploration into this concept, she began attending lectures at local meditation centers and universities on how meditation and spiritual practices can create a shift on a quantum level, which is to say down at the particle and wave level of the universe, the very base of existence. (Everything in the universe, a quantum physicist will tell you, is both particle and wave by nature.)

And since my mother had developed a personal philosophy that if something was helpful or meaningful to her, it should also be introduced to my sister and me, she began to take us with her to these lectures. At seven and nine years old, respectively, neither Harleen nor I always understood what these people were discussing; sometimes it just seemed plain weird. I remember one meeting in which we were each asked to bend the fork that had been placed on the table before us—they meant for the group to try to do this with their minds, but my sister and I, unaware of that part of the instructions, simply bent our forks with our hands. As the leader went around to examine what each person had done, he stopped abruptly at the bent forks sitting before my sister and me. Stunned, and perhaps believing he'd come across two young Jedis, he asked us to please teach them how we'd done it. "Easy," I said, and reached out to bend my fork some more. You could almost hear the deflation of hope in that moment!

Other lectures, though, did linger in my mind as a kid—particularly those that focused on the larger mystery at work in the universe, somehow linking everyone in energy and spirit. Later, when we were teenagers, my mother started to take my sister and me to meditation retreats. The first one felt as if she'd taken us to Paris after having studied French throughout our childhoods. We had become more fluent in meditation than we had realized, thanks to our mantras, and being given the chance to immerse ourselves in this world exclusively for a stretch of time felt expansive and revelatory in the best possible way.

Meanwhile, my mother had also begun to educate herself in Indian music and theory. She began playing different ragas, a type of ancient, often improvised classical music, throughout the day, each one meant to balance the energy of the environment at that specific time. In the evenings, when we were going to sleep, she would play the Samaveda, which contains some of the world's oldest surviving melodies, made up of Sanskrit verses meant to increase creativity and relaxation. For my eighteenth birthday, my mother sent me, along with my sister (for her sixteenth birthday), to a camp in the mountains of Northern California to learn about Gandharva Veda from the masters who lived in India. Gandharva (which means "skilled singer" in Sanskrit) Veda is a specific teaching from Vedic science about the influence of sound and music. These musicians and scholars taught me about how different types of Indian classical music are used to affect the body and mind and that Indian musicians were sometimes called upon to elicit changes in the natural environment such as to bring rain during a drought or even to fight natural disasters such as wildfires and storms.

Once, at 5 a.m., these masters, or Gandharvas, put on a concert—with only my sister and myself as their audience—in the forest. As they played, animals began to emerge, fluttering down from branches and peeking out from behind trees, drawn forth by the music. Birds, rabbits, even the skittish deer stood quietly and listened to the music. To this day, I can see the attentive poses and expressions of those animals clearly in my mind's eye; it convinced me of the possibility and significance in attuning oneself to nature through music.

My mother had not grown up with any of the Indian traditions she was now seriously practicing, but somehow they spoke to her from across the generations. She not only had felt immediately at home with them but also had an inherent confidence that they would benefit our physical and spiritual well-being. Of course, the irony of this development was not lost on my mother: Achieving the American dream had led her back to ancient India.

Meanwhile, I was on the path to achieving my own American dream. As my mother delved into these mystical pursuits, I doubled down on my schoolwork and ambitions. Though I did enjoy, and profit from, many of the experiences that my mother opened up for me, I also viewed them as separate from my primary goals. I was there to learn English, succeed at school, and become a professional. I was a straight-A student with straight-ahead ambitions. I had declared I would go into medicine when I was four years old. Despite my belief in my bija mantra, *my* culture was still about becoming as American as possible.

It was only when I went off to college that I began to glimpse just how second nature, and beneficial, the traditional Indian beliefs my mother had woven into our lives had become. As I started to get to know my classmates at Loma Linda University in Southern California, sitting with them in coffee shops and dorm rooms, discussing life in an adult way with people outside of my family for the first time, our conversations often circled the usual lofty topics of college students just finding their footing in the world: the meaning of life, the nature of reality. I found there was a major distinction between the others and me. I was drawing on the inner reality I'd cultivated throughout a childhood of meditation, while they were drawing on what they could see, hear, and touch in the world. In the classroom, when we were studying Western philosophy, we debated René Descartes's famous conclusion, ending his search for a statement that could not be doubted: "I think therefore I am." Yet I *did* doubt it. I *don't* think for large periods of time while I meditate, I told my professor, and I still exist!

I was able to assimilate opposing views, to bring together the mystic and the academic, whereas others often felt it was an either/or proposition. (It's perhaps not surprising then that I declared a double major of English and biology.) And, though I did well academically, it felt a little socially isolating to come up against this divide between my peers and me time and again.

I discovered my upbringing had made me an outlier in another way as well. Whereas my peers, finally out from underneath their parents' rule, would blow off steam or release stress by drinking a ton or doing drugs at parties, I realized I didn't feel I had anything to let loose *from*. With my mantra, I had cultivated a kind of "reset" button that allowed me to clear my mind and emotions twice a day, had quieted my fight-or-flight impulses, and kept stress from building up in my nervous system. Meditation had become as rote and essential to me as taking a shower; if I skipped it for a few days, I began to feel as if my brain were coated in a layer of grime, just as my body would feel if I hadn't bathed.

Once I reached medical school, however, the rigor and demands of my schedule made it challenging to keep up my daily meditation practice. The last three years of my neurology residency were the most difficult: An unpredictable schedule and brutally long work hours meant I meditated only sporadically. Those were, without a doubt, the darkest years of my life. I noticed a change in everything. I became more emotionally and psychologically fragile—which, frankly, is true of most medical students and residents—but I also felt more nuanced and intimate changes in myself. Where I had always been able to wash it all away no matter what had happened when I entered into that sacred, universal space, without regular meditation I felt out of control, trapped on the roller coaster of my moods. If I had a good day, I felt good; if it was bad, I felt bad. I was ruled by the physical world—and I realized for the first time that a large portion of humanity experiences life this way *all the time.*

I began my own clinical practice as a neurologist immediately after finishing my residency, in 2006. I was lucky enough to be given the chance to take over a successful neurology practice at Scripps Memorial Hospital in La Jolla, California, when the head physician retired. It was an unusual and tremendous opportunity: What most neurologists spend ten to fifteen years creating, I inherited from the start. This still meant working fifteen- to eighteen-hour days—but not having to build the practice from scratch meant I was able to completely give myself over to my patients, which I happily did.

But, six months into my newly realized version of the American dream, my own health began to plummet. And, like my mother, I found myself, for the first time, seriously debilitated by a condition. For me, this came in the form of crippling migraine headaches.

I tried to manage it myself with standard medication for about a year with no luck. So I consulted with a leading expert, someone who not only could offer invaluable advice but also knew me better than anyone else: my mother. She reminded me of the Ayurvedic medicine she'd exposed me to in my youth, which she had introduced to our family at around the same time she'd encouraged my sister and me to start meditating. This required that I change my diet, altering not only what I ate (avoiding processed foods, not combining certain foods, and adding turmeric, cumin, and coriander powder to just about everything, it seemed) but also *when* I ate, which was determined according to my digestive "fire," when the metabolism is more or less able to break down food (it is strongest at lunch and weakest at dinner). Also at my mother's counsel, I renewed my meditation practice.

My migraines vanished after three months.

My own experience reminded me—or perhaps it made me truly aware for the first time—of how effective these rituals had been for keeping my health in balance. And, of course, I'd long known that my meditation practice had kept me not only emotionally steady but also *connected*—to myself, to the universe, to a nourishing energy—throughout my life. How could

I have lost sight of that? And, more important, how could I not share these practices with my patients?

Two months after being headache free, I'd restructured my practice in order to offer integrative medicine. I started recommending—just as the American endocrinologist had done with my mother more than two decades earlier—that my patients see a meditation teacher and receive a mantra. I also began to prescribe herbs common in Ayurvedic practice, such as ashwagandha, for adrenal fatigue and stress; triphala, to support digestion; and brahmi, which can be beneficial to patients with addiction issues and many neurological conditions. I suggested that my patients take these alongside—or, when appropriate, instead of—prescription medicines. I even began to play Gandharva Veda, as my mother had done in our home throughout my childhood, as background music in the office to relax the nervous systems of my patients.

The results were stunning. Neurological problems are among the most difficult disorders to treat; the sad truth is that these are not patients who typically get better. In fact, in the short time that I had been practicing as a neurologist at that point, I had been dutifully prescribing medications and watching, helpless and frustrated, as my patients steadily got worse. That was the accepted convention of neurology: manage the symptoms as best you can in order to at least slow the decline. So when I saw people improving, one by one, using Ayurvedic medicine, I realized what my mother had arrived at instinctually: This five-thousand-year-old practice can offer more of an impact, in some ways, than modern medicine. We were, of course, an integrative practice—meaning we take into account the whole person and make use of all appropriate therapies—so I was happy to use Western medicine when it was necessary. But for many of my patients I found that with a shift in lifestyle practices according to Ayurvedic guidelines, they were able to slowly taper off of medications as their symptoms improved.

After we shifted our practice to integrative medicine, many of our patients struggling with epilepsy stopped having seizures; a number of people struggling with multiple sclerosis went into longer remissions, ultimately not experiencing another episode for more than a decade.

One woman, who was struggling with Parkinson's disease, came to us complaining that she was on too much medication and yet was not feeling any relief. She'd heard we had a different approach and she wanted to try it. We worked together for a year, slowly altering her habits—shifting her diet, giving her herbs, and having her start a mantra meditation practice—while also decreasing her medicine. By the end of that year, she was down to a very small dose of Sinemet, a medication that helps to ease the tremors, improve motion, and reduce rigidity of the body that accompanies Parkinson's disease, but no other pills. Previously, she'd been on four different medications, each at their maximum doses. Her physical abilities also vastly improved. Where she'd been hardly able to walk at all and spent most of her time in a wheelchair, she was now able to walk long distances with a cane. She was able to drive a car again. And, perhaps most important, she was able to go back to work, which not only helped her financially but also allowed her a crucial sense of purpose and fulfillment.

Of course, it wasn't as if we simply sprinkled some fairy dust and our patients instantly felt better. Some patients took as long as a year to fully change their diet or alter their sleep schedules. In the early part of the twenty-first century, the idea that our habits and lifestyle might alter our health was still up for debate, and many patients took time to trust in their efficacy. (These days, the principles of Ayurvedic remedies have become more widely accepted by American culture, but, believe it or not, there is still a large population of neurologists who don't accept, for example, that drinking water instead of soda may help reduce the severity of conditions such as multiple sclerosis.) Additionally, as a critical part of their treatment, I was asking many of these patients to start a serious meditation practice that included receiving a mantra. This is not a simple ritual to build; it takes time to create a routine, to trust your mantra, to take it seriously. On the other hand, many of these patients were in fairly dire circumstances, desperate to turn their health around, which can make a human as open as they'll possibly ever be.

Curious about the extent to which mantra meditation impacted my patients' recoveries, I decided to conduct an informal study with twenty-two of my patients suffering from multiple sclerosis. I chose this group because the progression of their illness is one of the most difficult to prevent; the lives of these patients—primarily women—were often halted by the disease at the height of their careers. Given, too, that it is clinically well known that stress can trigger MS flare-ups, these women were ideal candidates to try the anxiety-reducing tasks of Ayurvedic medicine. I also felt they'd be the most motivated to work with me on this, and I had a lot of compassion for them as well. Sixteen women made all of the lifestyle changes that we recommend based on Ayurvedic medicine *except* for practicing mantra meditation. The other six implemented all of the changes and were also sent to a Transcendental Meditation instructor who gave them each a bija mantra and helped them develop their practice. In studying the differences over the course of twelve months, my staff and I found that the disease progression slowed within the second group. Indeed, the MRI results of this second group actually demonstrated less inflammation and, therefore, fewer MS plaques. Additionally, when these patients did experience a relapse, they would bounce back more quickly and with fewer neurological symptoms. I concluded that the mantra meditation was allowing these patients to manage their stress better, which meant fewer opportunities to trigger a flare-up. This, for me, underscored what I had been increasingly coming to understand as a physician: Mantra meditation offers a significant defense against the inevitable stressors of life and therefore can create a bulwark against the advance of neurological disease.

In 2010, I was a guest speaker at an Ayurvedic course for health practitioners led by cardiologist Dr. Mimi Guarneri, who was, at that time, the head of the Scripps Center for Integrative Medicine. At the lunch, Mimi mentioned to me that she was about to leave on a two-week trip to India to visit with a spiritual teacher named Amma (which means "mother" in Sanskrit). As she told me more about this, I felt as if every cell in my body was firing at once, as if I'd just found the last piece of a confounding puzzle and was about to slide it into place. Over the years, my meditation has, I believe, honed my sense of intuition, and I've come to rely on it. The flashes of insight guide me both personally and with my patients, and my instinct very rarely leads me astray. But the physical intensity of the reaction I had in that moment was something on another order altogether.

I knew I had to go to India and meet Amma. Even if it would take me another decade to understand why I was doing something so impulsive, I knew in my soul that this was going to be a turning point in my life. To Mimi's astonishment, and frankly to my own as well, I bought a plane ticket for India that same day.

Two weeks later, we traveled to a small, rural town outside of Vellore, India, and set our bags down at Amma's ashram, a golden temple in the middle of a star-shaped path at the end of a single paved road lined by makeshift shacks selling fruit, clothes, and flower garlands. It was remote, but it wasn't quiet: As we approached the temple, we dodged oxcarts and rickshaws and motorcycles, not to mention a number of dogs scurrying about.

When I first met Amma, it felt as if I were walking back into a memory, though of course she, and this place, weren't attached to anything in my actual history. As we approached, her whole face broadened into a graceful smile and she generated more warmth and expansiveness than I'd ever encountered in a human before.

For the next five days, Amma and I, along with Mimi and twenty or so other devotees, went together to the pujas, which are spiritual ceremonies that take place daily. These ceremonies are *filled* with beatific sound. There is a cacophony of murmured

Vedic recitations; people are everywhere chanting mantras. At the end of each puja, Amma would distribute theertham, the water from the puja that had been "charged" by the mantras, meaning it had absorbed the energy generated during them. I felt an expansive energy there—it had a physical aspect in the sense that I sensed energy traveling up my spine, but I also felt an expansion of self and connection to others. Throughout this ritual, and in Amma's presence generally, I felt at peace in the same way I'd come to experience during meditation. In fact, it was so similar I felt as though I'd arrived at the physical manifestation of the place I'd been slowly building in my mind since I was nine years old. It felt familiar and momentous at once. Soon, I stopped wondering why I'd come and simply let myself be a part of it. Immersed in my own mantra meditation practice, I began to feel an expansion, as if my mind and senses were opening beyond my being. Which is to say I began to tap more freely into the universal energy field that connects all of us. I had evolved, it seemed, and deepened into the realization that I'd had as a child: There is a place within me that is also outside of me, where I am simultaneously my individual self and also self-*less*, at large and united with all in the universe.

I returned to California with a broader sense of meditation and its effects, not just for myself but as a doctor as well. I wanted to help patients find the same potent intersection of self and universal consciousness through mantra meditation. I had the first glimpse of what my genuine purpose might be and, as if on cue, my career began to take new form.

Since 2008, I'd been working to cofound New Practices, a company that would offer a new approach to health care management combining conventional medicine and integrative medicine through a research-based model. By 2015 we'd raised enough money from investors and our therapeutic model was sustainable enough that I stepped down from Scripps to become chief medical officer at New Practices. Around the same time, a producer from *The Dr. Oz Show* approached me about having me on as a guest to discuss the work I'd been doing as an integrative neurologist. Our conversations led to my first appearance as a guest on a TV talk show; ultimately, I participated in thirteen episodes with Dr. Oz, six of which focused on the chakras. During this time, I was also approached by the Chopra Center Mind-Body Medical Group—a pioneer institution in coupling Vedic science with modern Western medicine founded in 1996 by Deepak Chopra, M.D., and David Simon, M.D.—to work with them seeing patients a few times a week.

At the Chopra Center, I began to create a direct therapeutic relationship with sound for my patients. In addition to sending them to meditation teachers, I began to prescribe mantras for specific conditions, such as anxiety and depression, alongside traditional Ayurvedic supplements. I found that the patients who used the mantras recovered more quickly and required lower doses of herbs than the ones who relied solely on supplements. I also found that it wasn't just their health that improved. Mantra chanting added an introspective dimension to their recovery. Illness often carries with it a story; through mantra meditation, these patients were able to slow down and explore their own narratives, becoming more self-aware and realizing where they were stuck or blocked. This was a psychological expansion, certainly, but, on a deeper level, I believe they were also opening up energy centers in their bodies and allowing cosmic intelligence to flow through them.

In September 2016, I began to feel uneasy about New Practices. I had serious reservations about the integrity of some of the new investors joining the company. My hesitation grew exponentially over the following month; this culminated in my resignation in November. I had helped nurture this company for many years, and this was one of the most difficult decisions I have ever made in my professional career. I struggled with the weight of it, but in the end I chose principle over profitability.

Soon after, during my morning meditations, I began to feel a stronger and stronger call toward India and seeing Amma again. By this time, however, I had a husband and an eight-year-old child, and leaving to consult with my spiritual teacher, as I'd come to view Amma, was a much more difficult proposition. But this feeling increased during my meditations; just as a needle points toward the magnetic north on a compass, my internal needle was landing on India every time. Finally, in December 2016, I bought a one-way ticket to India.

When I stepped off the plane, I felt a sudden flash of fear that I'd gotten this wrong somehow; perhaps I'd permitted my desire to override my true inner voice. Perhaps I'd mistaken my yearning for intuition? But as soon as I saw Amma, a flood of relief came over me.

"How is your job, Kulreet?" she asked in her casual, all-knowing way.

"I quit," I said.

"Good," she said, and smiled.

And that was that. Suddenly, I had no schedule and nothing to do. For some, this might sound like a perfect vacation, but for me it was profoundly uncomfortable at first. I had been on a self-imposed schedule since I was in grade school. Outside of my meditation practice, I've made certain that my hours are always brimming with activity—I would fill even five minutes between meetings with something on my to-do list. Now, all I had to occupy my time was simply *being*. The phrase "being in the moment" is, these days, near ubiquitous, but, until I had no schedule in front of me and no return ticket back to a normal life, I had not adequately fathomed just what this really meant, or required.

After a couple of weeks of fidgety restlessness, I began to spend my days either in meditation, attending pujas, or in the deepest state of sleep I've ever had in my life. Some days I slept up to twenty hours. I also lost the sense of watching that I'd typically felt in my dreams. It felt instead as if I were simultaneously *in* the experience of my dream as well as outside, observing myself. The early Australian aborigines had an apt term for this state—*dreamtime*. They also believed this happened *everywhen*, a sort of time outside of time, and it was only when a person fell out of this state that he fell back into the narrow world of the present. In my own dreamtime, my senses felt more alive, everything shone with new luminosity, and, most crucially, the very fabric of space and time seemed to bend to the point that my sleeping, meditating, and waking lives all felt like one continuous reality.

After a month in this new state of awareness, Amma taught me to practice the chakra mantra, and my meditation practice expanded once more. I felt a profound sense of my body opening up; I felt fluid, less like skin and bones and more like the movement of energy. I began to see my connection to everyone and everything whether I was in or out of meditation. The world and everything contained within it seemed to have its own order. To come to this realization with the natural chaos of India as its backdrop—with cars constantly honking as pedestrians and stray dogs alike narrowly escape death while crossing the street—was particularly extraordinary. But there it was. I felt as if I had entered a school about the reality of the universe, and the answers to all of my questions came directly from experience.

Two months after that, Amma called me in to speak with her. We had not communicated since she'd advised me to meditate with the chakra mantra, so I was anxious to share my stories with her and to discuss my return to California. My husband and son had been patient for so long, and I felt it was time for me to move into the next phase, taking what I'd learned with me. I wasn't entirely sure what that next phase would be yet, but I also felt a serene confidence that it would come to me soon enough.

I went to Amma's home for lunch. When I arrived, I found her at a table turning over palm leaves, carefully examining each one. As I got closer, I saw that each leaf had something written on it. "What are those?" I asked, and then without waiting for her answer, I asked, "Are those the Siddha formulations?"

"Yes," Amma said coolly. "I just received them."

"Oh, by the way," she may as well have said, "here is the Holy Grail."

The Siddha medicine records are the most guarded tradition in India. The records, which are many thousands of years old, are recorded on palm leaves in an ancient Indian dialect and, for centuries, have been hidden in the temples of South India. As the leaves degrade over time, the information is etched again onto fresh leaves every 200 to 250 years by the yogis placed in charge of them. I first learned of these carefully guarded records when I'd begun seriously training in Ayurvedic medicine—I'd even tried more than once to access them myself. But I'd come up against the same challenge as every other person interested in these mysterious records: Nobody, it seemed, could get their hands on them, and even if it *had* been possible, they would not have been able to decipher them.

Amma turned another palm leaf.

I took a sip of my tea. Amma's composure had a way of laying a claim on everyone around her, so I sat there quietly transfixed.

She looked up again and asked that we go for a walk in her garden. As we ambled through the jasmine flowers, she asked if I would move to India and become the head of an Ayurvedic center that she was planning to build. "This is a family decision," she conceded. "But this could be the next step."

I felt joy and fear burst up at once from an unfamiliar place in me. It was as if she'd struck a chord so deep, I'd never even known the string existed. I knew that I had to slow down, to talk to my husband, to think about my son—but I also knew that I was not going to feel settled within myself unless I explored this possibility. Where I had once glimpsed just the outline of my purpose in life, I felt I was suddenly seeing it as a full, richly illustrated map.

I now live in India with my husband and eleven-year-old son. We've been here for just over two years, and in that time, I've helped bring the Ayurvedic center that Amma envisioned into being. It is a healing center—a place where we treat conditions from depression to arthritis to multiple sclerosis. We are also doing clinical trials and work with doctors at the nearby hospital who refer us patients with chronic conditions that are considered untreatable. We use spiritual practices as well—such as the puja ceremony and mantras—to "enliven" the herbs we prescribe as part of our therapies. Even the charged water from the pujas is offered to patients as a form of energy medicine. And, for the first time in history, the Siddha records are being translated for modern medical investigation. I am one of the first Western-trained physicians to study and implement the knowledge held in these records—an opportunity beyond my wildest imaginings.

One of the things that the Siddhas deeply understood about medicine was the healing capacity of sound. As I've come to learn, quite literally, every part of their curative practice involved sound. They had particular mantras, for example, to chant through every step of the production of the medicinal herbs they used—one mantra over the seeds, another for the growth, and still another for the harvesting and preparation. Sound was used to enliven certain qualities in the herbs and then later used as a tool for bringing health and harmony to the individual. Sound and mantra are in fact among the most essential part of the Siddha records, just as they have become fundamental to my own practice.

As I've immersed myself in mantra meditation here, both in my life and for my work, I have come to realize that I've been quietly and consistently studying these traditions for my entire life: as a nine-year-old practicing my first mantra and attending quantum physics lectures; as an eighteen-year-old in the forest listening to the Indian masters play from the Gandharva Veda; as a young medical student, when I learned more about the impact of my mantra meditation practice from its *absence* in my life; and finally as a doctor implementing sound therapy in combination with Ayurveda and Western medicine to powerful effect in my own life and the lives of my patients. There has hardly been a time, I finally came to recognize, when I *wasn't* immersed in mantra meditation.

I have made this inadvertent life study an explicit endeavor at the Sri Narayani Holistic Centre in India. As I've deepened my practice and knowledge of mantra, I've come to understand that its vibrational effect is also a portal into a much larger study of the healing power of sound. Modern medicine is still coming to grips with the potential of this discipline, but my own practice, through which I am able to connect to the deep silence within, has been a powerful guide as I straddle the worlds of science and ancient wisdom. Much of sound medicine draws from nature and the universal energy field connecting all of life; it is through mantra that I have experienced its profound impact on the human body and mind. As a doctor, however, I was eager to learn the scientific underpinnings of such a mystical and transformative practice.

2

THE BIOLOGY OF SOUND

There will come a time when a diseased condition
will not be described as it is today by physicians and psychologists,
but it will be spoken of in musical terms, as one would speak of a
piano that was out of tune.

—RUDOLF STEINER

The human body is designed to be exquisitely sensitive to sound.[1] In utero, our ability to hear develops by about eighteen weeks, making it one of the earliest senses to develop.[2] By the end of the second trimester, research has shown that a fetus responds specifically to the sound of a mother's voice and, once out in the world, babies demonstrate a continued preference for the maternal tone.[3] Doctors and hospice workers speculate that in the final moments of life, senses depart one at a time with hearing being the last to go—which is why we're advised to keep talking to our loved ones all the way through to the end, even after it seems they are no longer cognizant. Hearing is, in this way, one of our first and last modes of connection.

Though the sound that we imagine in these scenarios is something like voices or music, from a pure physics perspective, sound is silent. When we experience sound, what is actually happening is vibrations are passing through matter—be it a gas, fluid, or solid—in the form of a wave.[4] These longitudinal waves move by continually compressing and decompressing. Think of it like a Slinky stretched between two people: If one person gives her end a push, the Slinky ripples forward until it reaches the other person, then bounces back, continuing on and on. This compressing motion also determines the speed at which sound will travel. It takes longer for the sound waves to move through a less dense medium, such as air, because the molecules are farther apart, whereas in water, they are closer together and more quickly transmit the vibrational energy from one particle to the next, accelerating the speed at which the sound wave travels.

Vibrations transmitted as sound are measured in hertz (Hz), which captures the frequency with which vibrations occur every second. The middle C note on a piano, for example, is 262 Hz, meaning that there are 262 vibrations every second when that note is struck. By contrast, the fundamental frequency of a typical adult female voice—the lulling melody that we attune ourselves to in the womb—is 165 to 255 Hz, whereas a typical male voice is 85 to 180 Hz.[5]

It's astounding that we are actually able to hear the human voice at all when you consider *how* this happens. Our ears are an evolutionary adaptation that makes it possible for us to receive information from one person—who creates a pattern of pressure waves from the lungs that vibrate the vocal cords that then produce sounds—into meaningful speech. In order for these sound waves to make sense, we must transform sound waves into electrical impulses our brains can interpret. Once sounds pass your eardrums, these vibrations are sent to the middle ear, where there are three tiny bones—the smallest that exist in the body—called ossicles. These bones form a chain from the eardrum to the inner ear that transmits these sound waves to the cochlea, a snail-shaped structure filled with fluid and "hair cells," which are the sensory receptors of both the auditory (responsible for our sense of hearing) and vestibular (providing us with balance and spatial orientation) systems. When our ossicles move, the cochlear fluid begins to vibrate, causing the hair cells to shift as well. Different hair cells respond to different speeds of sound waves: Some move in response to higher-pitched frequencies, such as a baby crying, while others respond to lower pitches, such as a dog barking. The movement of these hair cells transforms the vibrations into electrical signals that travel via the auditory nerve—a bundle of nerve fibers running from the inner ear to the brain—where the information is decoded. Meanwhile, the auditory system also enhances useful information and reduces any distracting information from the various vibrations translating as sound from the world at large. Once the brain has finished deciphering this code, within about an eighth of a second, these vibrations become intelligible language while also indicating where the sound came from and in what particular tone of voice.

This is what happens *every single time* you hear a sound.

In addition to this complex transaction, vibrations can travel through our skin as well as the fluid[6] and bones[7] within us—just as they do through air—making our entire bodies strikingly receptive to sound vibrations.

In addition to this complex transaction, we are able to "hear" pressure waves through our skin as well as through the water that makes up roughly 70 percent of our body. And because water is less compressible than air, it conducts sound four to five times faster in our bodies. Last, sound can also be transported through our bones. In fact, our bodies are so conductive that physicians can use tuning forks to determine whether a patient has a bone fracture: A clear tone indicates an uninjured bone, whereas if the sound is diminished or absent, it indicates an interruption in the sound waves and the presence of a fracture is made known. Similarly, neurologists perform something called a Rinne test, which compares what we hear by air through the ear canal and eardrum to bone conduction through the mastoid bone to evaluate hearing loss.

There are also frequencies that are either too high or too low for the human ear to perceive, but are registered as vibrations through our nervous system. Though these vibrations are silent to us, they are still considered a form of sound, ranging from anything below 20 Hz, which are infrasonic frequencies, to above 20,000 Hz, which are ultrasonic frequencies. And, over the course of the last sixty years or so, these inaudible frequencies have become valuable mechanisms within the Western medical world.

The most prevalent example is the ultrasound scan. First used by an obstetrician in Scotland in 1956, it didn't become widely used in American hospitals until the 1970s.[8] These days, of course, the practice is now engaged to relay an image of the fetus to pregnant women, to examine internal organs such as the liver and kidneys, to reveal whether a lump is a tumor, and to investigate carpal tunnel syndrome, among other conditions. In an ultrasound, high-frequency sound waves—extending to 10 megahertz (MHz) and beyond[9]— are transmitted through a transducer, a wand-like probe that glides along the skin. These waves travel through soft tissue and fluids, such as blood, but once they hit something dense, such as a fetus, they echo, or bounce back. The deflection of sound waves hitting the transducer generates electrical signals that become an image, with varying shades of gray reflecting different densities.[10] Ultrasound is also used for therapeutic purposes by physical therapists and chiropractors, as it has been shown to increase blood flow, which can aid in tissue relaxation as well as reduce swelling, inflammation, and pain. It also stimulates production of collagen—the main protein component in soft tissues like tendons and ligaments—which can accelerate healing; these waves can even help repair bone fractures.

In 1994, doctors in Europe began using ultrasound for a noninvasive surgery known as magnetic resonance-guided focused ultrasound (MRgFUS).[11] Using a transducer, highly focused acoustic energy is pulsed into tissues in the body, which essentially heats up and liquefies unwanted growths such as uterine fibroids and prostate tumors.[12] (This surgery was approved for treating uterine fibroids by the Food and Drug Administration in the United States in 2004.[13]) The advantage to MRgFUS is that, since it provides such laser focus in treating a specific area, it doesn't harm surrounding tissue. Additionally, patients experience fewer side effects and need less time to recover than with more invasive procedures, such as surgery and radiation therapy.

In a similar way, infrasonic extracorporeal shock waves (inaudible frequencies on the other end of the spectrum, clocking in below 20 Hz) are used to break up kidney stones, ureteral stones, bladder stones, and gallstones in a treatment called lithotripsy. This procedure uses sound waves to target these stones and break them up into smaller pieces so that they can more easily pass through the body. Developed in Germany in the early 1980s,[14] this revolutionary discovery has allowed millions of patients with stone disease to forgo major surgery, which was once the only way to remedy this condition.

One of the most exciting uses of sound therapy is deployed in a procedure called high intensity focused ultrasound (HIFU). This is similar to MRgFUS in that it also precisely targets problem areas and disintegrates them with heat through an ultrasound probe. But HIFU uses lower, continuous frequencies to achieve thermal doses to interrupt faulty brain circuits— eliminating the need to drill or cut into the skull for surgery—or destroy unwanted tissue.[15] This system has been approved in Israel, Europe, Korea, and Russia to treat parkinsonian tremors and neuropathic pain, and has since been approved in the United States to treat essential tremor,[16] a neurological disorder that causes involuntary and rhythmic shaking, as well as uterine fibroids in women. There has also been promising research to show that this noninvasive therapy might also be effective in treating brain tumors, epilepsy, and breast cancer.[17]

In addition, in 2015, the U.S. Food and Drug Administration (FDA) approved two types of minimally invasive HIFU therapy, Sonablate and Ablatherm, for treating prostate cancer.[18] Although HIFU is a relatively new procedure in the United States, it has been used to treat prostate cancer in Europe for more than fifteen years with very positive results: an 86 percent five-year success rate for low-stage prostate cancer, with almost 80 percent of patients remaining free of cancer for seven years.[19] There are limitations: For one, HIFU is appropriate only for men with early stage prostate cancer with tumors located in a specific area within the gland; there are only a handful of surgeons in the United States who have been adequately trained to perform this procedure; and it doesn't yet have the long-term track record of radiation therapy or traditional surgery. And yet radiation and surgery both carry a high risk of undesirable side effects such as impotence and incontinence, whereas HIFU—applying hyper-focused sound energy—appears to offer a high success rate with little to no risk of these complications.

These are just a sampling of the promising developments inaudible frequencies have brought to Western medicine, and as a system we continue to make enormous strides toward harnessing sound waves to create immense health benefits. But there is even more to be gained as we explore the full scope of sound medicine and its astonishing power to heal.

The fundamental difference between the use of sound in Western medicine and alternative medicine is that the former relies on ultrasonic and infrasonic sound waves—inaudible frequencies—while the latter draws on vibrations that we can actually hear. There are, of course, a few exceptions to this rule.

In Western medicine, for example, there is a treatment called tinnitus retraining therapy that uses sound generators audible to the human ear to retrain the brain's relationship with the persistent unwanted ringing in a patient's ears so that it no longer affects them. But, for the most part, this is a reliable distinction between the two practices.

And yet when considering the ways we have evolved to be giant sound conductors—our skin, bones, ears, as well as the water that makes up a large percentage of our bodies all picking up sound waves—it makes sense that both inaudible *and* audible vibrations would have a profound effect on us.

In fact, recent research even shows that we pick up both audible and inaudible sound all the way down to a cellular level. In 2015, a study was published by biomedical engineering researchers from Columbia University building on the groundbreaking discovery that antenna-like structures containing an array of proteins on our cell membranes, called primary cilium, receive and respond to vibrational energy fields such as sound, light, and radio frequencies.[20] Primary cilia quiver like a tuning fork and, if a vibration in the environment resonates with the receptor's antennae, it alters the proteins' charges, causing the cell to change shape. This is a breathtaking discovery given that defects in the primary cilium have been linked to illnesses as wide-ranging as arthritis, polycystic kidney disease, obesity, heart failure, and cancer. And, if this structure is indeed receptive to such vibrational frequencies, the implication—one that is currently being researched—is that sound waves may have the capacity to reshape cell structures in a way that could help treat these illnesses.[21]

This is also the very principle that sound medicine is built on: When we are ill, the body's natural order of frequencies is altered, but when we are exposed to certain external vibrations in sound, our internal rhythms can be restored. This idea has been passed on through history from many cultures—ancient Egyptians, aborigines, Tibetan monks, Native American shamans, and Vedic masters among them. These groups have variously used chants, mantras, songs, and musical instruments to restore the vibratory frequencies of the body and mind, understanding instinctively what scientists were later able to prove: that there is a direct relationship between environmental sound and our physiological health.

You are likely familiar with some of the ways that sounds we hear can affect our heart rate, our breathing, and our brain waves. For example, when we hear an alarming or triggering noise—the sound of an ambulance or the explosive bang of a gunshot—the locus coeruleus (LC), a nucleus in the structure of the upper part of the brainstem responsible for mediating our physiological response to stress, is activated. Once active, the LC releases a flood of hormones, such as adrenaline, cortisol, and norepinephrine, into the body, initiating a string of other physiological consequences: our muscles tense, our heart rate increases, our pupils dilate, and our hearing sharpens. (The stress response, when originated in the LC, has in fact been found to be a major factor in stress-induced fear-circuitry disorders, especially post-traumatic stress disorder, or PTSD.[22] A 2005 study of American World War II veterans showed that combat-related PTSD is associated with a diminished number of neurons in the LC on the right side of the brain.[23]) This physiological cascade is also known as the fight-or-flight response, which evolutionary psychologists theorize developed in our early ancestors to provide them with a mechanism to act fast in the face of mortal danger. Today, this response occurs in humans not so much in the face of real threat but rather by more quotidian stressors, which means that it occurs more often but also fades more quickly.

By contrast, soothing sounds can have positive physiological effects.

When we experience sound waves either directly from or mimicking nature—such as waves lapping on the shore or certain bird songs—we relax. Research has shown that the sounds of nature increase attention capacity and shift our nervous systems into the rest-digest state.[24] Our breathing tends to slow, our heart rate decreases, and the nervous system releases oxytocin,[25] the so-called love hormone, associated with feelings of connection to others. And, when levels of oxytocin increase, other more arousing hormones, such as the stress hormone cortisol, decrease.

Though some of the notions of sound healing seem simply to be drawn from common sense—a serene piece of music will, of course, help you to feel calm—there is actually a complex interplay that occurs between external and internal frequencies. The two fundamental systems at work in this exchange are resonance and brain entrainment.

Resonance, which comes from the Latin word *resonantia*, meaning "echo," is an important concept in both physics and music theory. Broadly, resonance occurs when one object vibrates at the same natural frequency as a second object, thus forcing the second object to begin to vibrate. When one C tuning fork is struck, for example, and placed next to another C tuning fork, the second one will begin to vibrate at the same frequency as the first. In doing so, the sound wave from the first tuning fork has imparted some of its energy to the second one. And if the stem of the first tuning fork is placed on a metal, glass, or wooden object, this object, too, will begin to vibrate. This is also the metaphorical notion behind two people "resonating" with each other—this happens when a pair feels deeply connected and "in tune" with each other.

Similarly, every organ, every bone, and every cell in the body has its own resonant frequency. Together they make up a composite frequency for the body, as if they were each playing an instrument that, together, formed an orchestra. When one organ is out of tune, it affects the whole body. The goal, then, of sound therapy is to use audible vibrations to bring the body back into harmony and achieve what we call its "prime resonance" to restore health.

Once a person is brought into resonance, they are able to sustain this cooperative rhythm by entrainment, a concept that was first identified by the Dutch physicist Christiaan Huygens. Huygens invented the pendulum clock in 1656.[26] Almost a decade later, in 1665, Huygens discovered that when he set two pendulum clocks next to each other, they often became synchronized, creating "an odd kind of sympathy," as he once described it.[27] When the pendulum of each clock swings, it transfers a small amount of energy to the other clock. When out of phase, the waves of energy from each clock collide and produce negative feedback. In order to assume a more stable relationship, the amount of energy gradually equalizes with the object of a greater frequency slowing down, and the other speeding up.

We also see the law of entrainment in action when a group of birds fly in migration; they flap their wings together and glide at the same time to save energy, moving in a collaborative rhythm in order to take advantage of the pocket of air created by each bird in front of the other. It takes less energy for the birds to pulse in cooperation—and nature will always intuitively seek the most efficient functional state.

In the medical world, entrainment has come to describe a general shared tendency between physical and biological systems to coordinate their rhythms. The discovery of entrainment led researchers to explore whether or not the synchronous electrical activity of cortical neural ensembles—or, less formally put, the firing of brain cells—might alter and entrain their frequency in response to an outside sound. Brain wave entrainment, or more specifically neural entrainment, was indeed found to exist: The aggregate frequency of our brain cells can synchronize with that of an external source, such as the regularly repeating pattern of sounds or a sustained acoustic frequency[28]—which we perceive as rhythm or pitch. That is, our brain cells move in rhythm to the music that we hear around us.

The first music therapy intervention and systematic experiments were recorded in the early 1800s, though the notion that music has a healing influence appears in the writings of Aristotle and Plato.[29] Florence Nightingale was an early, albeit informal, proponent of using music to heal, having observed the

effects of different types of music on wounded soldiers in the
mid-1800s; "wind instrument pieces with continuous sound
or air generally had a beneficial effect," she wrote about the
response among her patients.[30]

Music therapy, however, wasn't widely brought into practice until after World War II, when musicians were hired to
play at veterans' hospitals around the country for veterans suffering from mental and physical traumas.[31] The response to
music—improving both the moods and health of these suffering soldiers—was so strong that hospitals started to bring
musicians on staff. As the need for people to train for this
burgeoning clinical profession increased, colleges began to include music therapy as part of their academic programs. Music
therapy gained in interest and credibility with the formation
of the Certification Board for Music Therapists (CBMT) in
1983, allowing for stronger credentials and the first music therapy board examination. In 1998, the American Music Therapy
Association (AMTA) was created, merging the National Association for Music Therapy (NAMT) and the American
Association for Music Therapy (AAMT), and has since become the single largest association for music therapists in
the world.[32]

At the same time, sound medicine has become a more vig-
orous area of research among scientists and researchers. Music
has been found to contribute to physiological changes in the
body such as the regulation of heart rate, pulse, blood pressure,
body temperature, skin conductance, and muscle tension; it
does so by sending a message to the more reflexive parts of the
brain that communicate with the autonomic nervous system,

which plays a central role in both inciting and quieting the fight-or-flight response.

Accordingly, music can both increase and decrease arousal in us. Multiple studies have shown that the amygdala—which is directly associated with feelings of fear and aggression—was active when subjects listened to music that was written in a minor key, was dissonant, or was just generally unpleasant. The amygdala's activity could even be modulated by a single chord change.[33] Listening to more pleasurable types of music, however, such as classical or jazz, has been shown to increase dopamine secretion, which is known as the "feel-good hormone" because it is associated with feelings of euphoria as well as a heightened sense of motivation and concentration. A 2015 study conducted by researchers in Finland contrasting participants who listened to Mozart's Violin Concerto No. 3 in G Major for twenty minutes with another group who did not listen to music for twenty-four hours prior to as well as during the study found that just twenty minutes of music enhanced the activity of genes involved in the secretion of the "feel-good hormone" as well as those connected with learning and memory.[34] (One of the most up-regulated genes was synuclein-alpha, or SNCA, which, when mutated, is the gene that is associated with Parkinson's disease. Interestingly, this is also the gene that allows songbirds to learn their songs.)

It may not come as a surprise then that music therapy has also been found to be helpful in reducing depression and anxiety.[35] Several clinical trials have shown that music has a positive effect on preterm babies with a beneficial impact on heart rate, behavioral state, oxygen saturation, and sucking and feeding ability, and decreases their length of stay in the hospital.[36] In 2008, Dr. Ronny Enk at the Max Planck Institute headed a study that discovered that not only did the stress hormone cortisol decrease in the three hundred people he'd had listen to fifty minutes of dance music but also their levels of antibodies increased, strengthening their immune systems.[37] A 2009 review of twenty-three studies covering almost 1,500 patients found that listening to music reduced heart rate, blood pressure, and anxiety in heart disease patients.[38] Along these same cognitive lines, a 2015 Stanford study showed that music engages areas of the brain involved with paying attention and updating events in our memory.[39]

Given that music communicates directly with the autonomic nervous system and stimulates hormonal activity, music therapy has been found to be especially useful in working with adults who have suffered some form of brain damage. In a 2009 study published in the *Annals of the New York Academy of Sciences*, researchers charted the effects of music therapy on people with traumatic brain injury. After administering just four separate thirty-minute treatments, researchers found that their subjects showed improvement in executive function—which allows for planning, organizing, and completing tasks—in addition to a decrease in depression and anxiety.[40] Similarly, but with a bit more specificity, researchers found in 2002 that adults with neurodegenerative diseases were helped in recovering lost memories by listening to Bach's Italian Concertos.

The fact that music can engage various and specific circuits in the brain also makes it possible to use it to modulate behavioral aspects in patients. Recent research has shown, for example, that music-based therapies can be beneficial for patients with Parkinson's by improving their gait—allowing significant improvement in speed and stride—and movement difficulties as well as reducing their number of falls.[41] This last finding also holds true for non-Parkinson's individuals. That is, music therapy has also helped to improve balance and decrease the risk of falling generally, a major risk for the elderly.

In 1980,[42] as this growing body of research was just beginning, a Norwegian teacher named Olav Skille noticed that when he had severely disabled children lean against a vibrating beanbag transmitting low-volume sound waves, they grew visibly calmer. Skille officially named this phenomenon Vibroacoustic Therapy (VT) and, since then, has done extensive research into the ways in which this process—applying low-frequency vibrations directly to the body, often in combination with selected music—benefits people struggling with a variety of conditions and symptoms including asthma, autism, insomnia, cerebral palsy, and Parkinson's disease.[43]

Since its inception in Norway, VT using "soundchairs" and "soundbeds" with loudspeakers built into them has spread[44] to Finland, Germany, Denmark, England, and Estonia, and it continues to be practiced with regularity throughout Europe. In 1997, an American study found that patients who had undergone open-heart surgery were able to reduce their hospital stay by an average of four days with postoperative sessions of VT.[45] It has since become a more popular practice in the United States, offered in spas and hospitals; the late Dr. Mitchell Gaynor, a distinguished Manhattan oncologist as well as founder and president of Gaynor Integrative Oncology, was a proponent of this therapy and used it to help cancer patients overcome the difficult side effects of radiation and chemotherapy.

Getting even more granular, there is also a body of research that explores the relationship between sound and our cells. Dr. James Gimzewski, a Scottish physicist and distinguished professor of chemistry at the University of California, Los Angeles, along with Andrew Pelling, a professor of physics at the University of Ottawa, has forged a new field in biophysics that he calls sonocytology. Using an atomic force microscope—which functions as a kind of super-sensitive microphone—to detect the vibrations of the cell wall, Gimzewski maps the pulsations of each cell's outer membrane and then amplifies it so that it is audible to the human ear.[46] This process has revealed that every cell in our bodies has a distinct sonic signature—its own unique song—as a consequence of its metabolic processes.

The "song" of each cell has the dynamic potential to interact with external sound waves and, Gimzewski and Pelling theorize, could be used as a diagnostic tool for identifying the sounds of healthy cells versus those of injurious ones.[47] This development would also introduce another, more dramatic, treatment frontier: the ability to play the destructive sounds of rogue cells back to them greatly amplified, so that they implode and are destroyed, not unlike the current use of ultrasound to break up kidney, urinary, and gallstones in lithotripsy. If this were implemented successfully, there would be no collateral damage to surrounding tissue, as can happen with radiation, since healthy cells would not resonate with these frequencies.

As a doctor who has extensively studied and practiced both Western and Eastern medicine, I believe we need to bridge the gap between the two in terms of their approaches to sound medicine, blending research and discoveries from both worlds in order to create a united and enhanced understanding of acoustic medicine. As a neurologist, for example, I never learned that sound actually alters proteins and changes cellular function; instead I studied how cells would respond to medication. Often research is done in a distinct discipline—the findings on sound vibrations shifting cellular function, for example, comes from molecular biology—but is not translated to other fields, such as neurology, within the world of medicine at large. This is, to a large degree, because medical practices—which operate far and away from the research departments of academic institutions and clinical laboratories—utilize only the treatments that already have a code for insurance to cover the cost. The health care system requires, in this way, that medical practitioners employ a myopic pragmatism as opposed to engaging with the dynamic discoveries occurring in medicine every day. In addition, an artificially divisive line has long been drawn between Western and alternative medicine as if one must necessarily be abandoned for the other—when, in fact, the two, taken together, offer advances in treatment that don't exist in one discipline alone. Even as I've moved to India, attended spiritual ceremonies, meditated in caves, studied the Siddha records, and started an Ayurvedic center, I've never left the Western world of medicine behind. This is quite literally true because I still practice in a modern allopathic hospital in India, but it is also true from a philosophical perspective. As mystical as sound medicine and mantra can be, I believe in uncovering the science and looking at the biological models to explain why and how any component works to sustain or restore our health. Although sound medicine as it was practiced by the ancients *is* beginning to reemerge in modern medicine—exemplified by the increasing number of hospitals and academic institutions, such as the Integrative Health and Wellbeing Program at Weill Cornell Medicine, that now incorporate sound medicine into their services—we haven't yet embraced the capability and dynamism of the human body and spirit. If, though, we can synthesize the evidence-based practice of Western medicine with the metaphysical concepts of ancient cultures and alternative medicine, we will be rewarded with stunning discoveries.

3

SPACE IS NOT EMPTY

Music gives a soul to the universe, wings to the mind,
flight to the imagination and life to everything.

—PLATO

Looking back on my life history, it makes sense that it has always felt effortless for me to move between the world of sound medicine—with elements drawn variously from ancient cultures and quantum physics—and the world of neurology, with its more intellectual, independent approach to the body. My early exposure to both Vedic medicine and quantum physics helped me to understand the dissonance between my inner reality—the timeless, disembodied realm of my meditations— and the external reality, in which I collectively took part at medical school and in the professional world.

Yet even with this particular ability to straddle both worlds, I still find it a challenge to wrap my mind around some of the more black-and-white models of science. In medical school, for example, I had difficulty with chemistry as well as classical

physics—not because I couldn't understand the principles, but
rather because I struggled to accept them as being ultimately
true. Some of the concepts stood in stark contrast to the way
I intuitively understood the world. When we learned about
how neurotransmitters worked with receptors, for example, I
was steeply challenged by the notion that all it took for a neurotransmitter to bind to a receptor—triggering the electrical
signals that inform our complex thoughts and rich emotions—
was for it to randomly slam into it. (When this happens, the
neurotransmitter "unlocks" the cell's response—giving rise
to the term "lock-and-key"—causing changes to it.) There is
something so inelegant about this idea, as if our thoughts arrive
on a system akin to bumper cars. It felt at odds with the sophisticated design of our brains; it just didn't seem a complete or
thorough enough explanation to me.

I also couldn't accept that the intense energetic connectedness
I'd encountered in my mantra meditations—the same energy
that had helped my patients to improve their health—should
be omitted from medical explanations to patients. I knew that
deepening our connections with our silent inner realities and letting go, if only temporarily, of the ping-ponging thoughts and
unchecked emotions we experience all day long had a measurable and dramatic effect, making me and my patients not only
physically and mentally healthier but also happier and more capable in our everyday lives.

The current Western model doesn't have a definitive, or
complete, explanation for what creates consciousness. We
know that too much or too little of a particular neurotransmitter can have a negative psychological outcome; we understand

that information from the brain is relayed to the body via the spinal cord and the peripheral nerves in the peripheral nervous system. But *how* our complex thoughts and emotions actually form is not accounted for in these mechanisms. I have come to believe that there is something missing from our understanding, something that would account for how our bodies receive and transmit information.

The answer to that question, and the way I have come to bridge the gap between physiology and consciousness, is a sense of spirituality. Before you mistake my use of this word to mean that I am trying to imbue medicine with religion, let me explain. In the Vedic tradition, the spirit is considered to be that which animates the body and gives us consciousness, as well as the ability to be aware of oneself in the world. It is the distinguishing mark of living things and our vitalizing force. Early Greek philosophers would have called this the soul, but you could also call it *qi*, as Chinese philosophy refers to this energy flow, or Brahman in the manner of the Vedic scholars. I do not believe there is only one right term; I mean *all* of these things when I refer to spirituality. If we don't take into account that which makes us living beings—that is, if we discount energy as a meaningful entity in medicine—we cannot comprehensively address our health.

In Western thought, quantum physics is uniquely reflective of energy's underlying and essential role in the universe; indeed this discipline describes nature at the smallest scales of energy levels. Throughout my studies, it has been a place of profound resonance for me, since it proposes scientific explanations, as well as a modern context, for the metaphysical revelations of

Vedic medicine. I believe that holding in mind both the sense of spirit proposed by the ancients *and* the rigor and research of science will allow us to open our minds to valuable and beneficial therapies, particularly in the realm of sound medicine.

Before we dive into the overlapping landscapes of consciousness and the quantum realm, however, let me take you back to the late 1600s, which is the juncture in history when we shifted as a culture toward viewing the elements of the universe as isolated—and as predictable and law-abiding as a machine. Sir Isaac Newton, the English mathematician, astronomer, author, theologian, and the father of modern physics—exerted a strong influence on this turning point. As the celebrated story goes, Newton first came up with the theory of gravity when he saw an apple fall from a tree—in the apocryphal version, the apple actually landed on Newton's head—and questioned the force that brought the fruit downward. "Why should it not go sideways, or upwards?" he reportedly asked, "but constantly to the earth's centre?" He went on to publish *Philosophiae Naturalis Principia Mathematica* (*Mathematic Principles of Natural Philosophy*) in 1687,[1] which included Newton's three laws of motion, describing the relationship between a body and the forces acting upon it, as well as its motion in response to those forces, thus laying the foundation of classical mechanics.[2]

Newton's theories explained both earthly and planetary motion, ushering in the downfall of the French philosopher René Descartes's vortex theory, which, among other things, proposed that the universe consisted of huge whirlpools of cosmic matter.[3] Where Descartes took a non-mathematical approach,

Newton's theories advanced from a mechanical, quantitative position.[4] Broadly speaking, the acceptance of Newton's model ended an era of philosophical speculation based largely on the theories of ancient Greek thinkers such as Plato and Aristotle and ushered in a more practical age of mathematically based experimentation as well as an absolute understanding of time and space.

Newton's view of the universe as a massive mechanical system revolutionized physics, but it had an effect on biology, too: From this point forward, doctors were trained to see the body as a machine, controlled by the brain via the nervous system, comprising isolated parts that malfunctioned in distinct ways, and without a sense of consciousness as a vital part of the whole. As a result, the medical community narrowed its view of illness; it became *only* about a single malfunctioning organ, divorced from any acknowledgment that consciousness—the complicated interplay of our thoughts and emotions as well as our energetic aspect, or spirit—might also play a role.

Newton's theories marked an astounding leap forward in many ways, but even as they led us toward much of our modern technological mastery, they led us further afield from understanding the life force that thrums in each of us, connecting us to each other and to the universe. Instead, our bodies were understood as machines that performed dutifully and predictably according to these new laws of nature. Western medicine is still largely governed by the belief that we must fix a discrete part rather than address the whole system—a myopic mentality that diverts us from addressing the real, or complete, problem.

In 1900, however, German physicist Max Planck countered

the theories of classical physics. He argued that energy occurs as a continuous wave-like phenomenon, independent of the characteristics of physical matter, suggesting that radiant energy is made up of particle-like components, known as *quanta*. The field of quantum physics was born,[5] and in 1918, Planck was awarded the Nobel Prize for his work,[6] bringing the discipline further into prominence. Other scientists, such as Albert Einstein, Niels Bohr, Louis de Broglie, Erwin Schrödinger, and Paul M. Dirac, advanced Planck's theory and helped to develop the theory of quantum mechanics, a mathematical application of the quantum theory that maintains that energy is both matter and a wave, depending on certain variables. That is, matter and energy are interchangeable forms. Quantum mechanics took a probabilistic view of nature, sharply contrasting with classical mechanics, which deals in precise properties of objects that are, in principle, calculable. Einstein, in particular, extended Planck's discovery by theorizing that energy itself—and not just the process of energy absorption and emission—is quantized. Light, he concluded, must consist of tiny particles called photons, and that certain phenomena could only be successfully explained if we took into account that both wave and particle exist in light. This is now known as the "wave-particle" duality theory.[7]

As the field of quantum physics took form and scientists began to look closely at the nature of matter, they also made some pivotal discoveries that were uncannily reminiscent of overlapping ancient concepts, such as those proposed in ancient Greek philosophy, Chinese medicine, and, of particular interest to me, of course, the Vedas. That is, quantum physicists, too, came to understand that there is a mysterious interconnectedness that exists and that a broader, universal energy underlies everything. This also marked the beginning of a slow shift toward investigating the links between energy, the body, and the universe and how these may be profoundly interrelated.

Yet quantum physics posed confounding challenges—even for some of its supporters. In 1935, Einstein, in a joint paper with Boris Podolsky and Nathan Rosen, put forth the EPR paradox, a thought exercise meant to show that quantum physics was an incomplete scientific exploration. This was, of course, a surprise coming from Einstein, who had been such an early advocate of and contributor to quantum physics,[8] even winning the 1921 Nobel Prize for his discovery of the law of the photoelectric effect, which is a quantum exploration of the nature of light and electrons.[9] But the renowned physicist had decided to withdraw support for quantum physics based, in large part, on the challenge it had come to present to his own work.

Einstein proposed the theory of special relativity in 1905 and then elaborated on it ten years later with his theory of general relativity. Simply put, the theory of special relativity explains how time and space are linked for objects moving at a consistent speed in a straight line. The theory of general relativity explored what would happen if acceleration were introduced to these circumstances and provided a unified description of gravity as a geometric property of space and time.[10] (Incidentally, Einstein's theory supplanted Newton's law of universal gravitation.[11]) For context here, however, it is important to note that Einstein's theory of relativity posited that an object anywhere in the universe is never able to travel faster than the speed of light. The measure of time under these circumstances exists in relation to how fast something is traveling in relation to the speed of light; in other words, time, in this realm, is relative. While the EPR paradox was meant to broadly demonstrate why quantum physics did not meet the deterministic requirements of a physical theory, it held a more specific, and telling, challenge within. Einstein and his colleagues laid out terms that disputed two essential quantum concepts: nonlocality and entanglement.

Nonlocality describes a phenomenon in which subatomic particles (particles smaller than an atom), when separated, behave as if time and space don't exist and are able to communicate instantaneously. This exchange between particles happens at a rate that is at least ten thousand times the speed of light.[12] This idea so outraged and confounded Einstein— who in his theory of relativity had established that the speed of light was the maximum speed for anything in the universe— that he simply refused to accept that this immediate transfer of information could take place. "Einstein Attacks Quantum Theory" a headline fairly screamed from the *New York Times* on May 4, 1935, above an article announcing that the famous physicist would appear before the American Physical Society to outline his criticisms.[13]

Still, quantum physicists forged ahead, propelled by this remarkable finding, and declared that nonlocality exists only because of entanglement, a phenomenon in which particles that have interacted with each other remain permanently connected, and are therefore able to continue to behave as a single entity even when separated by vast distances. For example, when a pair of electrons is created, one will typically have a clockwise spin, while the other will have a counterclockwise spin. Even if the pair becomes separated, when one begins to spin clockwise, the other will react by instantaneously spinning in the opposite direction.[14] Again, this occurs in violation of Einstein's speed of light law. Which may explain why Einstein later notoriously dismissed entanglement as "spooky action at a distance"[15] and steadfastly rejected nonlocality until his dying day, twenty years later, in 1955.

Nine years after Einstein's death, however, John Stewart Bell published a theorem—Bell's theorem—showing that all of quantum mechanics are intrinsically nonlocal.[16] Subsequent practical experiments have also proved that the effects of nonlocality and quantum entanglement exist,[17] verifying that "spooky action at a distance" does indeed occur.[18]

In the end, though, it was not just the threat these concepts posed to his own theory of relativity that Einstein opposed; he also felt a philosophical resistance to quantum physics, believing that it required too big a leap—and too big a paradigm shift. Nonlocality and quantum entanglement turned classic Newtonian physics on its head, proposing that everything is interconnected at the quantum level—the very root of life. But what if these quantum physicists also actually found evidence of the *spiritual* aspect of life and medicine that had once been proposed by the ancients? That is to say, what if these particles, separated by enormous distances yet always remaining connected, illustrate the oneness that is the central belief in ancient Eastern traditions and is the basis for their healing systems?

An essential concept in Hinduism—drawn from the Vedas—is the notion of Brahman, a genderless, bodyless energy; it is the ultimate reality, the source of all that exists. The Upanishads, texts from the Vedic era, define Brahman as "that which never changes; knowledge; infinity."[19] Brahman is also considered divine. As such, it cannot be described; it must be experienced. "Before they reach it, words turn back together with the mind," the Taittiriya Upanishad explains. "One who knows that bliss of *Brahman*, he is never afraid."[20]

Brahman makes no distinction between individuals. Through our connection to Brahman, we are made part of the whole—the oneness—that is being. Within the individual, however, exists Atman, a primal living energy sheathed within the body and mind. This is what we might call the soul or, in the sense that I referred to it earlier, the spirit. Atman, too, is eternal: When the body ends, Atman returns to Brahman. As in quantum entanglement, when two particles are joined, they are always linked. The concept of Brahman also suggests that the universe is a web of interconnection.

There is a related Vedic concept called maya, which, in the later texts of Vedic literature, means "a magic show, an illusion where things appear to be present but are not what they seem."[21] Maya extends from Brahman in that it proposes that the material world is an illusion. The separateness we perceive around us is a deception because we are actually unified by a profound, underlying force. Maya suggests that we create the material world because most of us are too unaccustomed, or afraid, to imagine ourselves as we exist in Brahman, without identity or boundary. Our reality, then, is based on a constriction of our consciousness. This constriction is also what drives us toward creating explanations for fragmented parts. So, for example, rather than seeing the body and mind as interrelated, we tend to see the individual organs and the lock-and-key model of biochemistry.

Nonetheless we are in contact with Brahman every day, and this shapes our lives in that it binds us to one another, whether we acknowledge it or not. If we are all entangled, as quantum particles are, then what each of us does affects *all* of us in some way (and giving profound meaning to the Golden Rule drawn from Jesus's Sermon on the Mount: "Do unto others as you would have them do unto you."). Relatedly, an essential principle of the Vedas is that the observer (what they call the rishi quality of consciousness) and the object of observation (the chhandas) and the process of observing (the *devata)* are interconnected, as they all arise from Brahman, the indivisible state of consciousness. Together, the rishi, chhandas, and devata make up the lila, which loosely translated means "the divine play," or the spontaneous creation of Brahman.

I believe, incidentally, that this sense of being both the observer *and* the observed is what I experienced in my pivotal visit to Amma in India when, sometimes sleeping up to twenty hours a day, I no longer felt I was simply watching my dreams, as a movie reel in my mind, but that I was simultaneously *in* them, experiencing them and watching them at the same time. Later, after Amma taught me to practice the chakra mantra, I began to feel my body opening up, as if I were more like the movement of pure energy. In those moments, I had, I believe, moved outside of my own consciousness enough to just touch

Brahman's subtlest edge, a field of bliss. My reality had shifted and I could sense some of the ways in which I was drawing from this vast energy source in creating my reality.

Interestingly, though perhaps not surprisingly, the notion of an unknown force playing a role in shaping reality—and, in particular, the belief that the observer, the observation, and the process of observing are interdependent—has also surfaced in quantum physics. Earlier in the chapter, I described wave-particle duality, the concept in quantum physics that everything at the subatomic scale must be viewed as both particles *and* waves. This was the first challenge posed by quantum physicists to our fundamental scientific understanding of existence. "We have two contradictory pictures of reality," Einstein once wrote, "separately neither of them [wave or particle] fully explains the phenomena of light, but together they do."[22]

There is, however, a finding that takes this one step further: The process of observation can actually *change* behavior within the quantum world. In classical physics, the experimenter is considered a silent observer. The universe carries on as it would regardless of this presence. But in the quantum world, there is a *relationship* between the observer and the observed, one that alters the fate of the quantum object.[23] This is called the "observer effect"[24] and is most often considered in relation to wave-particle duality.

The investigation that best demonstrates this mysterious phenomenon is called the double-slit experiment. In one version of this experiment, a series of photons (light particles) are sent toward a solid plate that has two parallel slits. On the other side, a photographic plate is set up to record what comes through these slits. If the photon passes through the slits unobserved—meaning there is no person or machine to measure its movements—it "interferes with itself," becoming a wave to travel through both slits at once. But if the photon, or particle, is being observed and measured, it remains the same, a particle, and travels through only one of the slits.[25]

In a twist that is reminiscent of the Vedic notion of maya, however, a series of experiments done by the physicist John Wheeler throughout the 1970s and 1980s showed that it was the sheer act of *seeing*, rather than any physical disturbance caused by measuring, that caused the photon to change form. In his "delayed-choice" experiments, Wheeler used a clever series of beam splitters timed to measure the paths of quantum particles *after* they should have chosen whether to take one path or two. As it turned out, it made no difference whether the measurement was delayed or not: The result was the same. That is, as long as the photon's path was being observed before its arrival at a detector, it did not become a wave. The very notion of being seen, then, made the particle behave consistently as an observer might expect it to be.[26]

Wheeler's finding has sparked all manner of controversy and debate within the scientific world, undermining as it does the very foundation of science—that is, the assumption that there is an objective world, irrespective of us. But, as the double slit experiment seems to illustrate, if how the world behaves is dependent on the observer, and the process of being observed, we are living in, as Wheeler himself once called it, a "participatory universe."[27] It would seem this quantum finding corroborates the Vedic notion that we create, and shift, our lives based on our subtle communication with Brahman, or a vast energy source.

Throughout history, both philosophy and science have touched on a universal field of energy—as well as how our relationship with it might work. In Vedic philosophy, there was the belief that, whereas Brahman is the unmanifested energy of creation, Akash is the first manifestation of life in the form of vibrations: where life comes to life, so to speak. Vedantic Hinduism proposed that four elements arose from Akash; these, in the order in which they emerged, were air, fire, water, and earth. Akash, too, was believed to be a substance, although not atomic in nature; it was seen as an all-pervading energy that fills space. Like Brahman, it was formless, infinite, indestructible, and incomprehensible to the ordinary intellect given its divine nature, although it contained energy in motion in the form of vibration (as opposed to the pure, potential energy of Brahman).

And each of these elements, according to the Vedas, is associated with a sense: Touch is associated with air; fire is connected to sight; water is correlated with taste; earth is linked with smell. Akash, the subtlest form, is linked with hearing. In this sense, we're participating with the universe through our mind and five senses. And since the Vedics believed hearing was the first and most essential perception given its link to the Akash, then sound was the first line of communication with this vibratory aspect of life.

Held within the Akash, Vedic philosophers perceived, were

the Akashic records, a field that records all that has happened in the universe. This was considered the compendium of all human events, including every thought, emotion, and intent that has occurred in the past, that is occurring in the present, and that will occur in the future. This field was also the medium through which the vibratory nature of Akash could pass and be made evident in life. It is also within the Akash, it is believed, that the divine and primordial sounds of nature are "recorded" as vibratory codes and were interpreted by the Siddhas as mantras.

This is why mantra meditation is so vital within Vedic philosophy and Siddha medicine: Chanting a mantra is a deliberate act with a specific, prescribed intention for outcome. The thoughts in our minds, according to Vedic philosophy, are also sound, and therefore if you are able to have thoughts with intention you are communicating your desires and manifesting your life more directly into the vibratory substance of the universe from which all matter arises. Even silent mantras, when chanted in the mind (and provided that they mimic the primordial sounds of nature, as all of the Vedic mantras do), still act as sound waves and can alter the vibrations within the body. As such, Vedic philosophy believed—and the Siddhas were adeptly trained in this—that mantra meditation was a precise way of participating with the universe.

Akash is also the Sanskrit word for "atmosphere" or "ether,"[28] which points to the progression of our implicit understanding of the Akash through history. For example, ancient philosophers such as Aristotle and Pythagoras believed, just as the Vedantic Hindus did, that there were four elemental conditions—air, fire, water, and earth—that arose from a fifth element, the *quinta essentia*, or quintessence, which they called ether.[29] Unlike the four other elements, ether, they believed, was boundless and indestructible. Sound familiar?

Descartes brought the idea of ether into the scientific realm in the seventeenth century with his aforementioned vortex theory, in which he rejected the notion of a void and proposed instead that space was filled with a subtle substance that was the carrier of force and light.[30] He, too, believed, as Vedic philosophy originally suggested and the Greek philosophers carried forward, that this was a primordial substance, infinite and infinitely divisible.[31] Later, Newton (who, you'll remember, overturned Descartes's vortex theory with his three laws of motion) described a density-varying ether that could provide a mechanism for gravitational attraction.[32] With Newton, ether became a widely accepted notion; among physicists, it became known as a space-filling substance, a medium that allowed for the propagation of electromagnetic or gravitational forces.[33]

By 1913, however, quantum physics had proposed a new version of ether—and another explanation for the subtle material capable of holding and transferring energetic vibrations, which they called the zero point field, or ZPF.[34] As the theory goes, about 13.7 billion years ago in the first fractions of a second of the Big Bang, when the universe was born from a single point in space, there were no particles of matter, but rather virtual particles.[35] Virtual particles, in quantum physics, occur when one particle becomes a pair of heavier particles that then quickly rejoin the original particle, as if the pair had never existed at all.[36] These virtual particles, in the time that they fleetingly appeared, exchanged energy with other quantum particles, causing erratic fluctuations of energy. This subatomic exchange, amazingly, still takes place today; throughout the history of the universe, these particles have been continuously popping in and out of existence in the vacuum that was once considered ether—and before that, Akash.

Zero-point energy is the vibrational energy that molecules retain even at an absolute zero temperature.[37] In physics, "temperature" is a measure of the intensity of molecular motion; zero temperature is the moment all molecules come to rest, yet there is still a flurry of measurable activity. So it is the energy of the ground state of any system; everything has a zero-point energy, even a particle cooled down to absolute zero will exhibit some vibrations.[38] These vibrations, it is believed, are contributed to by the activity of virtual particles coming in and out of existence. What we have essentially understood space to be is not empty at all but rather the collective ground state energy of all the fields in space, or what is known as the zero-point field.

"If you add up all the particles in the universe constantly popping in and out of being, you come up with a vast, inexhaustible energy source—equal to or greater than the energy density in an atomic nucleus—all sitting there unobtrusively in the background of empty space around us, like one, supercharged backdrop," says Lynne McTaggart, author of *The Field: The Quest for the Secret Force of the Universe*.[39]

In other words, what we once held to be vacuous is in fact teeming with vibrations. The entire universe is literally singing with energy.

Quantum physicists have proposed that the ZPF, or the "field of fields,"[40] as it is sometimes referred to, is constantly interacting with all of the subatomic particles of the universe; the movement of one drives the other forward. This repository of energy thrums throughout, consistently emanating vibrations and subatomic waves.[41] An important aspect of these waves is that they encode information in the form of energy and they have a virtually infinite storage capacity. So if all subatomic matter in the world is interacting constantly with the ZPF, the subatomic waves of this field are constantly creating a record of this activity. In this sense, the ZPF serves as a kind of memory for the universe—which sounds remarkably similar to the Akashic records.

More than any other field in modern science, quantum physics offers the strongest link to the ancient Eastern traditions and systems of knowledge, particularly Vedic philosophy and Siddha medicine. And whether you call it the ZPF, or Akash, or spirit, there is more evidence than ever before of the ineffable oneness and energy connecting us to each other and the universe. In this sense, we can look to the past to understand our future. As a result of the scientific inquiry quantum physics has opened, we're starting to see the emergence—or, rather, *reemergence*—of vibrational medicine. In essence, we are circling back once more to the concepts of Vedic medicine and Siddha tradition.

4

THE HUMAN BIOFIELD

We have now discovered that there is no such thing as matter; it is all
just different rates of vibration designed by an unseen intelligence.

—PHYSICIST MAX PLANCK, UPON ACCEPTING
THE NOBLE PRIZE FOR PHYSICS IN 1918

Not long after I'd started to run my neurology clinic at Scripps
Memorial Hospital and decided to practice integrative medicine, I began taking a course to further explore Ayurvedic practices. In this class, I learned to take the pulse of my patients in
a particular way: I put my index, middle, and ring fingers on
the inside of a patient's wrist and, by applying varying amounts
of pressure, determine the vata (related to the Akash and air),
pitta (related to fire and water), or kapha (related to water and
earth) balances—the three doshas that make up the vital energies of the body.[1] Each of these provides a blueprint for a person's mental and physical health; to a skilled practitioner, they
are used to ascertain the constitutional type and energetic balance of the body as well as the overall well-being of the patient.

When I implemented this routine in my neurological practice, however, a startling thing began to happen. I started
picking up additional information about my patients. When
I would take a patient's pulse, seeking this technical aspect of
the Ayurvedic diagnosis, I would also get an instinct about the
person's emotional state. At first, this was subtle enough that I
almost didn't recognize it—or perhaps it was so unfamiliar, it
was hard for me to discern that I was getting a flash of someone else's feelings. Sometimes the information would come in
the form of a picture, other times I would hear something in
my mind. I began to get a picture of their lives with specific
details about childhood traumas or whether a family member
had fought in a war or the current state of their relationships. It
wasn't that I was psychic or having visions; it didn't feel spooky.
In fact, it felt clear and practical, as if these stories were as
empirical, and necessary, to knowing about a patient's health
as taking their blood pressure or listening to their heartbeat.
These feelings became sharper and more delineated until I finally realized I was actually navigating my patients' mental and
emotional terrains. I would know if someone was feeling depressed or anxious; their emotions would come over me as if I
were experiencing them myself, but with enough distance that
I didn't feel personally distraught.

In this way, I was briefly able to try on my patients' thoughts
and emotions, and it gave me a tremendous sense of empathy.
But I also felt extremely uncomfortable, as if I were reading a
personal letter meant for someone else. I was shy and cautious
about what I was gleaning, and at first I didn't mention it to
anyone at all. Slowly, though, as more and more information

came through—and I became aware that I was cultivating a valuable awareness for my patients—I began to disclose what I was experiencing. More often than not, my patients would respond by asking me how I could discover something so intimate about their lives simply by taking their pulse.

I remember, in particular, a woman I'd treated as a patient from the beginning of my time at Scripps. She was a lovely woman, always pleasant to my staff and funny and gregarious in her visits with me. Once, when she came to see me, not long after I'd finished the Ayurvedic course, I put my fingers on her wrist to take her pulse and was abruptly taken aback.

"Oh my gosh, you're so angry," I said, surprising myself with the informality of my own comment. But I had felt a completely unexpected and astonishing rush of fiery temper. The woman stared at me for a long moment, during which I wondered if I'd inexorably overstepped my bounds. "How did you know?" she finally asked. As it turned out, she and her husband had been struggling for a long while and were seriously questioning whether they should stay together. They'd also had a blow-up just before she'd come to visit me.

This ability to sense my patients' interior worlds through pulse has only deepened for me since I've moved to India and begun my work with Siddha medicine. It's as if I can peer into a tunnel, glimpsing patients' lives when they were fourteen years old, six years old, sometimes ten months of age. I saw someone the other day and, as I held my fingers to her wrist, caught sight of a place that I knew—and *felt*—used to tie her stomach in knots when she walked by it. Every time I meet with a patient it is an incredibly intense experience, and it creates a profound bond for both of us. I also enter a state similar to what I feel when I meditate: My thoughts disappear, my mind becomes silent, and, in the moments before I get a flash of insight, everything is completely still. Once I do start sensing the mood or memories of a patient, I feel immersed in the same serenity that washes over me during meditation as well. I feel enormous compassion, too, as if there were no separation between us.

This feeling of oneness, I believe, comes from tapping into a universal energy field—the place in which we are all connected; what the Vedic scholars call the Akash and what quantum physicists refer to as the ZPF. This broad energy field touches everything. Just as the Vedic masters believed four primary elements (air, fire, water, and earth) emerged from the Akash, I believe that there are also fields emerging from this reservoir of all the vibrational movement of life that surround our bodies—these are what are known collectively as the human biofield.

The notion of an energy field spans all disciplines, of course, from classical physics to quantum physics to the newer model of biofield science. In classical physics, a field refers to a nonmaterial element, or an invisible region, that connects points in space and can extend infinitely.[2] This was what Newton meant when he proposed the concept of a gravitational field, a model he used to explain the influence that a massive body extends into space around itself, producing an attractive force on another massive body. Contemporary physics holds that there are only four types of force operating throughout nature: gravity, electromagnetism, and the strong and weak nuclear forces (these last two have a range limited to the atomic nucleus).[3] Our understanding of the electromagnetic field in particular has evolved over time so that now we know that this field is not just a way of calculating the force exerted on another object but also a space through which energy can be transmitted, even within the human body.

The electromagnetic field is what is used in conventional medicine to measure the electrical activity of the heart and brain. Medical doctors track this vibrating field of the brain with an electroencephalogram, or EEG. Our brain cells communicate using electrical impulses; an EEG analyzes the brain's activity and sends signals to a computer that records the results—these are the wavy lines, creating peaks and valleys, that you see on the computer screens in hospitals. Doctors use these recordings to detect any irregularities that may be causing specific brain disorders, such as seizures. The heart, however, produces the largest rhythmic electromagnetic field of any of the body's organs—roughly sixty times greater in amplitude than the electrical activity generated by the brain—making it the most powerful source of electromagnetic energy in the human body.[4] The heart's electrical field is measured using an electrocardiogram (ECG or EKG for short). Doctors can use this record to track the heart's rhythm; detect the blood flow to the heart; diagnose a heart attack; and check on anything that may appear abnormal, such as thickened heart muscle.

In discovering that there are measurable electromagnetic fields created by the human body—as Nobel Prize–winning doctor and physiologist Willem Einthoven did in 1901 when he invented the prototype for the ECG machine[5] and German psychiatrist Hans Berger did when he created the EEG in 1924[6]—it became imaginable that other fields might exist in the body that we hadn't yet acknowledged.

In fact, we have the work of prominent Russian biologist Alexander Gurwitsch, alongside Hans Driesch and Paul Weiss, to thank for the notion of the biological field that informs our medical practices to this day. The mystery of how the embryo develops in such a coherent and dynamic manner—which endures today—captured Gurwitsch, who once wrote that this "miracle" had "determined the direction of all my research work."[7] For the first half of the twentieth century, he developed his morphogenetic field theory, proposing that the morphogenetic field (also referred to as a biological field or biofield) offered a causal link between the individual parts of the embryonic process and may explain the highly organized developmental process of the human embryo. In his work, he studied cell division in the embryonic process of sea urchins, chicks, and onion roots and asserted that this field was an organizing force behind cellular division patterns during mitosis.[8] Weiss, in particular, determined that this field remained unchanged even after removing portions of embryonic tissue and also suggested more broadly that the biological field served as an organizing principle for the entire body.[9]

Interestingly, the actual word *biofield*, the shortened term for biological field, was not officially coined until 1992, when the Office of Alternative Medicine at the U.S. National Institutes of Health (NIH) convened an ad hoc committee of complementary and alternative practitioners and researchers to discuss their work. In their discussions, they realized they needed a universal term to apply to the complex organizing energy they were proposing was engaged in the generation and regulation of health.[10] The biofield also reincorporates the ancient concept of a vital force, which the ancient Eastern healing traditions, as well as their related energetic therapies, are founded on. The formal definition for biofield given at that time was "a massless field (not necessarily electromagnetic) that surrounds and permeates living bodies and affects the body."[11] Yet Dr. Beverly Rubik, a biophysicist whose career focus is the subtle energetics of living systems and, incidentally, one of the congressionally appointed members to the Office of Alternative Medicine at the NIH who instituted the term *biofield*, aptly describes it as "nature's original wireless communication system."[12]

The discipline of biofield science has expanded since, aiming to elucidate and provide a scientific foundation for energy therapies such as acupuncture, Reiki, therapeutic touch, qigong, and, of course, sound healing. Biofield scientists and the practitioners of its energetic therapies strive to understand how such a field might interact with the body and why the alteration of it can affect our health. Biofield science also takes into account aspects of the whole being—physical, psychological, and spiritual—as opposed to the constricted view of its discrete parts.[13]

This does not mean, however, that biofield science is practiced at the exclusion of—or in renunciation of—conventional medicine. On the contrary, the primary aim of this science is to create a fuller, more comprehensive medical system. "While each view has its limitations, together they are complementary, similar to particle-wave duality, the principle of complementarity in quantum physics," Rubik wrote of the advantage of such a merger in the *Journal of Natural and Social Philosophy*. "Together they offer a more comprehensive view of the living state. Life is simply richer and more complex than it is possible to express in a single model or metaphor."[14]

Intriguingly, a variety of Eastern traditions—Tibetan Buddhism, traditional Chinese medicine, Siddha medicine, and Ayurvedic medicine, among them—created systems acknowledging the biofield as they understood it and describing concepts related to it in terms of achieving health. The Vedic texts, specifically the Taittiriya Upanishad, likely composed about sixth century BC,[15] offer a sophisticated and richly detailed cartography of how energy flows through the body, charting the pancha kosha—the "five bodies" or "sheaths" as translated in Sanskrit[16]—believed to enfold a person. These sheaths (what Western scientists would call "fields") surround the individual sequentially, making up a person's biofield; each sheath serves as a veil obscuring the underlying universal energy field, or Brahman, that is the true nature of all human beings. As each successive field becomes closer in proximity to Brahman, it grows in its power to shift the energy of the human body. In other words, altering the energy of an inner sheath affects all of the sheaths that are more superficial to it. Each is related to one of the five elements (ether, air, fire, water, and earth) that make up the universe. Each one also has a name ending in the word *maya*, which, as you'll remember from the last chapter, means "magic show," but in this context refers to "creation," as in the illusory creation projected from Brahman. Together, these fields offer a map for the connection between individuated consciousness and a broader field of energy; each one offers a new depth at which human life operates.

The most superficial sheath is the annamaya, which is associated with the physical body, essentially the blood, bone, and skin. *Anna*, in Sanskrit, means "food," suggesting that this layer reflects the tangible, physical body. If we live exclusively identifying with annamaya—as many of us in the modern world do—we will identify with the physical body alone. This, too, is the sheath that mainstream medicine tends to investigate because it is material. In this sense, Western medicine mainly concerns itself with 20 percent of the human biofield, thereby limiting its repertoire of solutions to suffering and illness.

The second field is pranamaya—*prana* being "life force" in Sanskrit—which surrounds annamaya. Pranamaya both vitalizes and links body and mind, manifesting physically in breath. As long as prana exists in the body, life continues. This is the energy field, according to Vedic philosophy, that has the capacity to heal through the flow of prana; it can be reached by energy therapies such as Reiki and acupuncture. Sound therapy, too, has an effect on this field, but since sound is generated as vibrations from within Akash, it also has an impact on all the subsequent fields. Vedic medicine also identified a complex network of pathways in the body, called nadis (the root *nad* means "channel" in Sanskrit[17]), through which prana flows. Nadis are similar to the acupuncture meridians of traditional Chinese medicine; the body is crisscrossed with 72,000 paths accessed through the subtle energy body of the pranamaya. It is worth noting that Tibetan Buddhism also describes a network of 72,000 invisible energy channels.[18]

The third field is the mind sheath, manomaya, which is the source of the five senses (hearing, touch, sight, taste, and smell) and the ego. This field guides our thoughts, emotions, memories, and decisions. It is also what leads us to cling to our individual identities and stands in the way of a full awareness of Brahman, or the underlying Self. Mantra meditation, incidentally, is the most powerful tool to quiet this field, which is vulnerable to the fluctuations of all that we perceive and process daily in our minds through our senses.

The fourth sheath is known as the wisdom sheath, formally called Vijñānmāyā, comprising the discriminating intellect, which discerns between what is real and what is not, what is maya and what is the true nature of reality. Although the actual mind tends to pull our attention toward the physical body and the material world, the wisdom sheath draws awareness toward the Self. It digests and analyzes incoming sensory impressions received from the outer mind—the manomaya kosha—and extracts meaning from it. However, our fears and judgments from the mental sheath can cloud the knowledge body's ability to distinguish between the real and the unreal. This sheath is also the source of electromagnetic fields within the body, and as you pierce this sheath, knowledge of the subtle fields of matter becomes apparent to you. When Vijñānmāyā is unburdened of the clutter and noise of our minds, it is possible to access the wisdom of Brahman or the Self. This opens a person to extraordinary intuition, wisdom, and objectivity. I believe when I am taking the pulse of my patients, the insight and details of their lives come to me because I have reached this point in myself and therefore am able to access information held within their collective biofield. It is in the wisdom sheath, too, that one can start to comprehend the interconnectedness of the observer, the observed, and the process of observing. Upon reaching this level of consciousness, I have come to profoundly understand, as Shakespeare once deftly put it, "all the world's a stage, and all the men and women are merely players";[19] we are actors, all of us, collaborating in a divine drama.

Which brings us to anandamaya, or the "bliss" sheath, where consciousness and the vibration of energy first meet. Anandamaya is the vibratory energy from which all the other sheaths arise; it is the last layer of individuality surrounding the Self, and the subtlest part of our own creation, which draws from the eternal silence of universal consciousness. This field is the seat of sound. The waves generated from the vibrations of the universal energy field can be perceived by humans through sacred sound—such as a mantra meditation—and when these vibrations permeate the denser fields and begin to resonate, a person begins to connect with the divine energy of Brahman. This is what is considered enlightenment in the East.

The ancient Eastern traditions developed theories similar to some of the discoveries taking place in science and medicine today. The ancients used introspection—as opposed to machines such as the EKG or EEG—to measure the body's biofield, but the goal of Vedic medicine intersects with that of the contemporary and emerging field of biofield science: to actualize the considerable powers we have to heal. Unfortunately, modern science allows for only a limited recognition of the biofield, focusing its investigation on what the Vedics would call the annamaya kosha, or the physical body. The discovery of measurable electromagnetic fields surrounding the heart and the brain has pushed modern science beyond its traditional focus on the material and physical body, but we are only beginning to understand pranamaya, the vital principle that connects the body and mind, from a Western perspective.

It is here that biofield science has taken up the reins, combining the knowledge of Eastern traditions with the tools of modern science in an effort to heighten our knowledge of the fields that remain imperceptible to us. It is more useful to speak of these fields in terms of their effect on the body—their influence on a variety of biological pathways including biochemical, cellular, and neurological processes—than as actual detectable entities. To that end, Jacques Benveniste, the late French immunologist who came into prominence in the late 1970s as part of the research team that isolated the blood-clotting protein called platelet-activating factor (PAF), conducted experiments that are crucial in understanding the ways in which we might explore and understand biological field effects.[20] In 1984, Benveniste was studying the reaction of certain white blood cells to allergens.[21] After an accidental dilution of the allergen, one of Benveniste's lab technicians recorded a reaction in the white blood cells even though there had been too few molecules of the allergen physically present in the water to make this happen. Intrigued, Benveniste repeated the experiment several times, always arriving at the same conclusion: The vibration of molecules, the smallest particles in a chemical element or compound, can be "recorded" in water so that they need no longer be physically present to effect a result.

Benveniste published his finding in *Nature*, one of the world's most prestigious multidisciplinary science journals, in 1988, along with thirteen other scientists who had replicated the results in four different laboratories in France, Israel, Italy, and Canada. Despite the preexisting replications of the experiment, John Maddox, then-editor of *Nature*, took the unprecedented step of arranging for an independent follow-up investigation. This group failed to replicate the original results,[22] a scandal that prompted Benveniste to defend his method in letters published in *Nature* that explained the protocols used in the follow-up were not identical to his own.[23]

Based on his research and that of his colleagues, Benveniste maintained that, when dissolved in water, a substance acts as a template, altering the electromagnetic properties of water.[24] In subsequent dilutions, the properties of the substance dissolved in the original solution are transferred to newly added water, demonstrating, as one journalist dubbed it, "water memory."[25] This challenged the quantitative structure-activity relationship (QSAR) theory, which states that when two molecules of matching structures meet, they exchange specific chemical information.[26] That exchange occurs when the molecules bump into each other—the very same lock and key interaction model that I had felt so challenged by in medical school.

His findings, though, left unanswered an essential question: Where is this memory being held? The inherent concept of Benveniste's experiment is that the molecule itself was no longer the source of the information—how could it be? It is no longer present in the solution—yet the field in which it once existed contains that memory in waveform and is capable of transferring that coded information directly to water—sounding remarkably similar to the idea that the Akashic records hold information within the waves produced by vibrational energy.

Benveniste continued to test his hypothesis that the signaling between molecules was not biochemical but, rather, occurred through low frequencies, which are within the range of the human ear and thus produce sound. He developed experiments using a computer to record the signature frequency of certain molecules and then used an amplifier to play back the frequency alone to a biological system.[27] In doing so, he made the case that he could "fool" the biological system into thinking it was interacting with the substance using only the sound of the frequency of the molecules. Benveniste even went one step further by testing the "sound" of an actual medical drug, the anticoagulant medication heparin. Heparin prevents plasma, the yellowish medium of blood, from clotting, even in the presence of calcium—which can be used to control clotting capacity by removing it from the plasma and then adding back in certain amounts of the mineral. For his experiment, Benveniste removed calcium from the plasma and then added it to water. Then he exposed the water containing calcium to a digitized electromagnetic frequency of heparin.[28] The sound had the same effect as the molecules of heparin itself would have. Again, this suggests the biofield effect in action, illustrating that a transfer of vibrational information through sound can have a tissue effect.

Amazingly, Benveniste's work is a kind of precursor to the sonocytology research created by James Gimzewski. Together, Benveniste and Gimzewski offer a penetrating look at how sound is the underlying foundation of all biology. Another way of seeing it: By using sound to alter the vibrations of the deepest field—the anandamaya kosha, as a Vedic scholar would explain it—you affect all the subsequent sheaths, including having a biological effect on the tissue in the body.

Similarly, Beverly Rubik, who you'll remember as the biophysicist who helped coin the term *biofield*, conducted a study published in 2006 attempting to quantify the effects of Reiki treatments, a Japanese healing technique performed with the hands to move energy in the body. To eliminate the placebo effect—the idea that a beneficial result is produced by the beliefs of a patient—Rubik took patients out of the equation altogether,[29] and instead asked Reiki practitioners to administer treatments for fifteen minutes on heat-shocked bacteria. As heat shocking would result in the death of many of the bacterial colonies, the experiment was designed to investigate, in an impartial way, whether Reiki had an observable physiological effect.

The practitioners treated the bacteria in both a healing context (meaning they had treated a pain patient for thirty minutes beforehand) and a nonhealing context (there was no treatment of a pain patient beforehand). No overall difference was found between the control (untreated bacteria) and Reiki plates in the nonhealing context. In the healing context, however, the Reiki-treated cultures displayed significantly more bacteria than the controls, indicating that the bacterial colonies that had been eliminated by the heat shocking had regenerated and recovered. Furthermore, the initial level of well-being of the practitioners (determined by questionnaires administered before and after all sessions) also correlated with the number of bacterial counts, suggesting that the contentment—and connectedness, too—of the practitioner has an objective effect in treatment.[30]

As I've mentioned, it is known that there are measurable electromagnetic fields around the heart and brain—and both are widely used for diagnostic purposes in Western medicine. More recently, a wealth of research has been done on the heart-brain connection and how these two organs, through their vibrating fields, are in extensive communication with *each other*. The focus of much of this research has been on heart rate variability (HRV), which is the naturally occurring beat-to-beat variation in heart rate. Though it was once thought that the heart at rest was like a metronome, beating at a steady and regular rhythm, it is now understood that the rhythm of a healthy heart is surprisingly irregular, with the time interval between beats continuously changing. HRV, then, measures these variations in heart rate from one beat to the next.[31]

HRV is governed by the relationship between two branches of the autonomic nervous system (ANS)—the sympathetic nervous system and the parasympathetic nervous system. The sympathetic nervous system accelerates the heart rate in response to stress or fear as part of the fight-or-flight response. The parasympathetic nervous system acts as a decelerator, bringing the heart rate and body back to physiological balance. The regulation of the heart by the autonomic nervous system is well known, and well documented; however, as a 2014 article published in *Frontiers in Psychology* with more recent data, from studies ranging from 2006 to 2012, suggests, "a more complex modulation of heart function by the intrinsic cardiac nervous system"[32] may also be at play. This cardiac nervous system is comprised of independently operating intercardiac neurons, leading some researchers to characterize it as the "little brain" in the heart.

The sympathetic and parasympathetic nervous systems are continually interacting, all day long, with the aim to keep cardiovascular activity within its optimal range. HRV reflects the stability of the system as a whole and is regarded as an important gauge not only of health and fitness but also of physiological resilience and behavioral flexibility. In other words, HRV indicates our ability to adapt to stress and environmental demands. The factors that influence our HRV include breathing patterns, exercise, and especially our thoughts and emotions— one of the most dynamic contributors to altering the heart's rhythm is emotion.

Accordingly, chronic stress and related emotions such as anger and frustration alter HRV so that the rhythm patterns become erratic, rendering the HRV waveform a series of jagged peaks. This pattern signals that the two branches of the ANS are out of sync with each other, unable to work cooperatively in order to calm the body down after a heightened cycle of negative emotions.

Conversely, positive emotions such as appreciation, joy, care, and love cause the heart rhythm pattern to become highly ordered, looking like a smooth, harmonious wave. This is called a coherent heart rhythm pattern. When our hearts beat in a coherent rhythm, the sympathetic and parasympathetic nervous systems are synchronized. The stable pattern of the heart's input to the brain both eases cognitive function and bolsters emotional stability. This means that learning to generate increased heart rhythm coherence by sustaining positive emotions not only benefits the entire body but also profoundly affects how we perceive the world around us.[33]

The HeartMath Institute, an organization founded in 1991, committed to exploring the interdependent relationship between physical, mental, and emotional systems, has done intriguing research on how stress, intuition, and human energetics affect heart-brain interactions.[34] Where it is commonly known that the brain sends neural signals to the heart, the HeartMath research shows that the heart sends even *more* signals back to the brain, which has a significant effect on brain functions such as attention, perception, memory, and problem solving.[35] Studies conducted by HeartMath have demonstrated that when the heart rhythm pattern is erratic and disordered, the subsequent pattern of neural signals traveling from the heart to the brain actually inhibits higher cognitive functions, limiting our ability to think clearly, remember things, learn, reason, and make effective decisions. The heart's input to the brain during negative emotions also has a measurable effect on the brain's emotional processes, reinforcing the experience of stress. Similarly, these incoherent patterns of physiological activity can deplete our energy and produce wear and tear on the entire system. This is especially true if negative emotions are prolonged or experienced often.[36]

This cutting edge research on HRV underscores that we experience emotions first physiologically, in our bodies, and *then* interpret them in our brains.[37] By learning to control our hearts, whether through deep breathing or meditation, we can gain mastery over our brains—and vice versa. These findings have significant implications for biofield science, supporting the idea that the electromagnetic fields surrounding the heart and the brain interact in such a way that affects our health; the heart actually *shifts* brain wave function through a field effect. Furthermore, the way that the heart and brain come into resonance, as measured by an EKG and EEG respectively, during periods of sustained positive emotion, is an example of the heart entraining the brain. As the fields of the heart and brain vibrate at the same natural frequency, they are able to sustain a unified rhythm. What is so astounding to me about these findings is that resonance and entrainment—cornerstones of sound therapy—occur naturally between the heart and brain. It would seem that entrainment happens as a function of our mental state, suggesting that a field effect transpires between the emotions and heart and brain.

Indeed, in a series of recent preliminary studies, it has been found that improving HRV in a variety of people struggling with cognitive disabilities, ranging from combat veterans with post-traumatic stress disorder[38] to clinically stable patients with schizophrenia[39] and patients struggling with severe chronic brain injury,[40] has helped each of these groups, respectively, with attention and memory issues; anxiety and stress; increased self-awareness and self-esteem; and regulation of emotions.

Despite the promising work coming out of biofield science, however, this discipline faces a steep uphill battle to finding its place in conventional medicine, even with an integrative model beginning to gain a foothold. Though conventional medical clinics and hospitals such as my own former hospital, Scripps Memorial, the Cleveland Clinic, and Johns Hopkins Hospital have made substantial investments in order to offer integrative medicine to patients and staff, my fear is that Western medicine will simply assimilate the more acceptable aspects of biofield science—fitting this new information into its existing models and understanding as it has with acupuncture and music therapy—rather than reshaping perceptions to accommodate the entire field.[41] For biofield science to become a mature paradigm, its research and evidence must be taken seriously, and it must be allowed to dismantle preexisting notions of the medical establishment when its findings are strong and consequential enough to overtake an old way of thinking. The medical system must be flexible, developing its capacity to adapt, or we stand in our own way of making meaningful progress.

The first, and most difficult, hurdle that biofield science faces is that it is inherently anomalous within the conventional medical paradigm because the research is not based on a recognized, material biological mechanism but rather on the subtle, and largely undetectable, movement of energy within fields.[42] This is made only more complex by the assumed connection to religion within biofield science and among its related healing therapies—despite the fact that its researchers and practitioners have reinterpreted these ancient Eastern traditions in secular ways. There is, of course, a *spiritual* aspect to biofield science, as it acknowledges that our consciousness plays an inextricable role in our health, but this by no means stipulates any one dogmatic approach. Whether you find quantum physics or Eastern traditions, or, as I do, some combination of both to be a useful framework, in order to develop a system that addresses the whole being, we must take into account the roles of energy and consciousness.

The crux of this conflict is apparent in an exchange that took place in 1999 on a panel at a conference about complementary and alternative medicines.[43] Marcia Angell, then-editor of the *New England Journal of Medicine* (*NEJM*), participated on the panel and fielded a question about editorial bias against findings from the alternative medicine world. Angell responded that, in order to be "good" science, a study must offer a plausible biological mechanism for the effect reported, otherwise the study was not believable. She then offered several examples of alternative medicine studies—including a study of moxibustion, an Eastern medicine practice that is a form of heat therapy, for breech presentation—and declared that, despite sound statistics and clear results, these findings "could not be true," because they failed to present an acceptable biological mechanism. Therefore, they should not, she concluded, be published. Ironically, the moxibustion/breech study *had* indeed already been published in the well-respected and peer-reviewed *Journal of the American Medical Association* (*JAMA*).

In his classic 1962 book, *The Structure of Scientific Revolutions*, the philosopher of science Thomas Kuhn, who himself revolutionized the way we look at patterns in scientific progress, made a distinction between *normal science*, that which belongs to a prevailing model and is about "puzzle-solving" or contributing new information to an established structure, and *revolutionary science*, which involves a revision to the existing scientific belief or practice. There is a great deal of resistance when it comes to revolutionary science, as it requires a paradigm shift and, in some cases, an intimate revision of our beliefs—recall Einstein's reaction when quantum physics posed a steep challenge to his theory of relativity. Scientific anomalies are often ignored or explained away so as not to disrupt a well-established order.

But Kuhn also made another, perhaps more productive, point about how science might successfully move forward, even in the face of threat and defiance: He asserted that there must be a strong commitment within the scientific community to shared theoretical beliefs, values, techniques, and *metaphysics*—what Kuhn referred to as a "disciplinary matrix." He hoped that this matrix would allow for the open pursuit of all questions within science, including the mysterious anomalies—a transformation that, on its own, would be a scientific revolution.[44]

As a medical community, we must open ourselves to knowledge outside our siloed disciplines and beliefs. I am a neurologist, yet I see every patient that comes through the hospital where I work in India. Every physician has a specialty at this hospital except for me. I am known as a doctor and a healer and, now that word has gotten around, "the lady who can see inside of you when she puts her hands on your wrists." Even in the United States, I was a bit of an eccentric; I saw the patients who nobody else could "fix."

As a direct result of my role here, I recently started an addiction therapy program to help treat alcoholism, a disease that affects some 60 percent of the population in the region of India where I live. Because it is such a prevalent and virulent problem, both the hospital and patients have been open to my taking this over because they don't know what else to do. As with indigenous populations worldwide, many struggle because they are not as educated on the dangers of alcohol and have turned to drinking as a balm for the many traumas inflicted on their culture throughout history and from living in poverty today. I believe, too, that the people I am treating may lack the genetic structure, as has been found in many of the indigenous peoples, that allows them to effectively break down alcohol, which means alcohol converts to sugar rapidly but is not taken out of the bloodstream as quickly.

In our work with these patients, I, along with a team of three other doctors, am helping them to create a regular mantra meditation practice; we are complementing that practice with herbs to normalize the response to dopamine receptors and shift the "reward center" in the brain from craving alcohol. We've also encouraged them to enroll in Alcoholics Anonymous. The program is still too nascent for official results, but, anecdotally speaking, this multipronged program has yielded many positive results.

The trouble is, if this program is a success—as I suspect it will be—there is not a place in the current medical biological model for me to offer a study on why a combination of mantra, herbs, and counseling could have a significant effect on something as difficult to control as alcohol addiction. I don't have a language to talk about this with my colleagues in the United States—and even with many of my colleagues here at the hospital—because there isn't a world yet in which we can believe in this.

Ultimately, I share Kuhn's hope that we will reach a moment where modern medicine can open itself and accommodate all aspects of biofield science—that we can integrate, as I do, the deep wisdom of Eastern metaphysics and the rigorous inquiry of Western medicine. Biofield science needn't be perceived as a threat. We don't have to choose one model over the other. We simply need to open up to the presence of this new paradigm so that we might fully address the abundance and range of possibility in the human experience.

5

THE CHAKRAS

Our own physical body possesses a wisdom
which we who inhabit the body lack.

—HENRY MILLER

In 2018, about a year after Amma had taught me the chakra mantra, I felt a strong inclination during my daily meditation to record myself chanting and share it with others. It was an odd message to receive given that I was accustomed to silently repeating the chakra mantra during meditation; it felt foreign to utter it out loud. Moreover, I am quite shy about my voice and have always avoided singing in public—which is essentially what I would have to do if I made this recording. But I'd come to trust these directives, even more so after the chakra mantra increased the sense of my own consciousness ebbing and flowing, as it did, from the universal energy field. And I felt certain it would be worthwhile to follow my intuition.

I asked my husband, Joshua, to accompany me in this undertaking. Unlike me, he has a beautiful voice. We decided we would each sing on our own and then combine the tracks in editing. We set up a little recording studio in a closet in our house, where I could hide from the world as I chanted. As testimony that I'm not just being self-deprecating when I say I am not a good singer, before we began, Joshua asked only half-jokingly if I wanted to do a short prayer for my voice before we began recording.

To both of our astonishment, when he pressed the record button and the words ushered from my mouth, I sounded wonderful! When we shared the recording with family and friends, they were equally amazed. They encouraged us to post the recording on iTunes, which we agreed to do. A few days before our iTunes debut, however, I received a call from a producer for *Megyn Kelly Today*—this was when the program was still in its early stages, only a few months after it had premiered and nearly a year before its unhappy ending. The producer said they were interested in doing a segment on chakras, ideally something that might be interactive with the audience—did I have any ideas? I don't know how the producer got my name, or my cell number for that matter, but her call did not surprise me.

Let me interrupt my own story here to say I know how eerie, perhaps even unbelievable, this turn of events may sound. As I say, I no longer feel that way about it given how often these kinds of things happen to me—but I have not lost sight of the startled feeling I had in the beginning, when a thought or an inkling would come to me in meditation and then, soon enough, would materialize in my life. But I have also developed a confidence that relating stories like this is part of my aim, and responsibility, if I am going to successfully create a bridge between the known scientific world and the more mysterious realm of Vedic medicine. I stand firmly with one foot in each world—as both are consequential—and it's important to me to help others see the advantage in understanding both modern and ancient disciplines in a complementary way.

And so on January 17, 2018, I sat onstage with Megyn Kelly and led her studio audience, as well as her 2.4 million viewers,[1] in the chakra mantra chant: "Hari Om, Nam Lam, Mam Vam, Sim Ram, Vam Yam, Yam Ham, Shiva Om, Swaha," I intoned as Megyn Kelly gamely chanted alongside me. And we kept on going through the commercial break. There was a strong and exhilarating energy in the room. At the end, Megyn leaned over and whispered, "I don't know what all that was about, but I definitely felt it." We had, it seemed, just balanced Megyn Kelly's chakras.

Chakras are a concept that many are familiar with but few truly understand. Where Western medicine tends to view human beings as a collection of organs held together in a single physical sheath, Vedic medicine considers the body to be composed of five sheaths. These sheaths—which collectively make up the biofield or energy body—collect and transmit information that the chakras translate into physical phenomena in the body. I like to think of the biofield as the software and the chakras as the hardware on which this information is downloaded.

As a neurologist, I learned that the spinal cord is a pathway for information to flow from the brain to the body. The cord is filled with nerves that send electrical signals between the brain and organs. As an Ayurvedic practitioner, I learned that each chakra—which means "wheel" in Sanskrit,[2] symbolizing dynamism and movement—functions in a somewhat similar way to the nerves. This system, which originated in India several thousand years ago and was embraced by many Eastern traditions,[3] including Buddhism and Hinduism, encompasses thousands of chakras in the body—each one existing at a dense energy center where the nadis, the network of 72,000 pathways running throughout the body, intersect. Interestingly enough, there are major bundles of nerves that run along the spine that correlate closely to where the majority of the chakras are located. The seven main chakras run from the base of the spine to the crown of the head, and our emotions, physical health, and mental clarity—all guided by the information being relayed from our biofield—dictate how much energy is emitted from these chakras into various regions in the body.

I knew about chakras growing up, of course, but in the same superficial way that most people know about them: I understood from my mother that they were an essential part of Vedic medicine, that they existed in the body and had something to do with our health. But when I began to receive detailed information about my patients by taking their pulse, I also began to see patterns between certain medical issues—be it asthma or depression or Parkinson's disease—and how each of these expressed in the energy body. Curious, I dove into the Vedic texts and research on chakras and my instincts were confirmed: These energy centers were a vivid and detailed map to my patients' ailments. If I find problems in a particular organ,

I know now there is an associated sheath in the biofield where I will find corresponding physiological and psychological issues as dictated by the chakra system. In other words, chakras are animated by a dynamic blend of consciousness and anatomy and facilitate the energy that runs through the body's biofield.

Just as the Vedic tradition asserts that each of the five elements—ether, air, fire, water, and earth—is associated with a particular sheath of the biofield, so, too, are they related to certain chakras. This creates a repetitive pattern: The five elements are associated with five sheaths of the human biofield and the first five of the main chakras (the last two chakras are considered to be in the spiritual realm and therefore not affiliated with one of the five elements). This synchronous, layered organization common in Vedic philosophy has since been found by modern mathematicians to be true in nature as well as within our bodies. Such a pattern is called a fractal, which recurs at progressively smaller scales, so that every part of it resembles the whole. Perhaps the most amazing discovery about fractals is that they are infinite in surface but finite in volume; the pattern can go on forever but is contained by its own design. We see spontaneously occurring fractals, large and small, in the jagged shapes of lightning bolts, the eddying waters of a stream, and snowflakes. Additionally, our neurons and even our lungs are fractals—which is how, in the case of our lungs, the body packs the surface area of a tennis court into a rib cage.[4] In nature, there is an abundance of fractal organization and behavior, though it is admittedly less iterated and precise than the mathematical fractal.[5] Still, objects like ferns and seashells maintain an extraordinary intrinsic coherence.

Essentially what the fractal design illustrates is that nature keeps repeating its own pattern, on a micro and macro scale.

This is true, too, of the five sheaths and five chakras as they reflect the five elements. To give an example: The water element is related to the pranamaya sheath, the site of entrance for the creative life-giving force, prana, and the sacral chakra, characterized by flow and flexibility[6] and associated with the reproductive organs and the urinary system (both of which have an overt connection to water) as well as sensual pleasure and creativity. As we'll soon explore in detail, the five elements also repeat with the doshas so that we see how Vedic philosophy espoused—and in a sense predicted—the idea of fractal organization in the subtle energy body as well as the physical body.

I had known intuitively as an Ayurvedic doctor that these centers needed to be unblocked when energy wasn't flowing through them freely, but as my understanding of chakras came more distinctly into focus, I realized how crucial this process was to my patients' overall well-being. Chakras are like tubes that can get clogged by stress or fear—these types of menacing emotions create a blockage, along with environmental pollutants or an unhealthy diet. Opening up the chakras is like flushing this tube of its waste and debris. The ultimate aim is to activate all of the chakras, so that they are all in balance and open and allow the energy of the Self to permeate the body to its fullest extent. This balancing is most effectively achieved through sound—specifically chanting the chakra mantra. Though I am still working toward activating all of my chakras on a continual basis, I have experienced moments of complete opening. This is what happened when, as I described early on, I began to feel my body become fluid, more like pure energy. Indeed, I see my own mantra practice divided in two: before Amma taught me the chakra mantra and after. I believe, too, that this mantra has helped many of my patients access this universal energy. But before we dive into the mantras themselves, let's take a brief tour through the seven chakras and the role they play in our bodies and lives.

THE FIRST CHAKRA
THE ROOT CHAKRA (MULADHARA)

Located at the base of the spine, right at the start of the tailbone, this first chakra corresponds to the earth element and the annamaya kosha, what Western medicine considers the physical body. It is correlated with basic survival needs, such as food and shelter. When it's balanced, we feel grounded, safe, secure, and connected to the earth's energy field. People blocked in this area are more likely to experience emotional issues surrounding money and security. They will also feel decreased vitality and increased fatigue. Since the root chakra is also associated with the large intestine, rectum, and adrenal glands, blockages in this chakra are also more likely to result in physical problems like lower back pain, fatigue, and GI problems such as diarrhea or constipation. Emotional signs of an underactive chakra include feeling fearful or nervous, while signs of an overactive chakra are expressed in materialism and greed. Energy from this chakra propels upward to energize all of the other chakras.

THE SECOND CHAKRA
THE SACRAL CHAKRA (SVADHISTHANA)

This chakra, located in the lower abdomen just below the belly button, is the seat of our creativity and is connected to the water element as well as the pranamaya sheath. As I mentioned earlier, this is the chakra where prana is brought into the body, and it also guides our sexuality, creativity, and emotions. A balanced sacral chakra allows us to take risks or be passionate, sexual, and outgoing. It also allows us access to the unconscious mind and, as such, work on this chakra often releases blocked or obscured emotions. When it is not able to channel energy properly, we may experience a creative block or trouble with relationships. When it is overactive, we tend to react with exaggerated feeling to everything. Since this chakra is associated with the reproductive system—the testicles, uterus, and ovaries (in Vedic medicine, the reproductive organs are also considered the creative organs)—health problems associated with this chakra include infertility and sexual dysfunction.

THE THIRD CHAKRA
THE SOLAR PLEXUS CHAKRA (MANIPURA)

Your third chakra is located in the hollow area where the ribs meet above the belly button. Correlated with the fire element and the manomaya kosha (the mind sheath), this is the seat of the mind and ego. Many of the longings of the ego erupt from this chakra, but, as one evolves spiritually, a more universal desire develops—the desire for right action and outcome. This chakra also controls motivation, ambition, self-esteem, and willpower. When it's balanced, we are able to act fairly yet assertively and set appropriate boundaries. Alternatively, people whose solar plexus chakra is blocked tend to have poor self-esteem and self-control and struggle with issues such as codependency. When the third chakra is overactive, it tends to make people domineering and aggressive. This chakra is also associated with the organs of digestion—the liver, gallbladder, stomach, spleen, pancreas, and small intestine—putting people at higher risk of developing nutritional deficiencies and other gastrointestinal problems like gas, IBS, bloating, and stomach ulcers when it isn't functioning properly.

The gut-brain axis is perhaps one of the most familiar and evidenced systems in Western medicine. Beginning in 2004,[7] a series of studies described the biochemical signaling that takes place between the GI tract and the central nervous system, indicating a link between brain health and the gut microbiome. This echoes the ancient Vedic view of this chakra, which governs the organs of digestion and is connected to the mind sheath.

THE FOURTH CHAKRA
THE HEART CHAKRA (ANAHATA)

This fourth chakra is of particular importance because it's at the center of all seven chakras—with three above and three below. Located in the center of the breastbone aligned with the air element and the vijñānāmāyā kosha (the knowledge body), this is thought to be the chakra where the physical and spiritual intersect. "Within the heart there is a luminous consciousness which is intelligent, imperishable, and effulgent," as it is described in ancient Vedic scriptures. The heart chakra is the source of a loving, compassionate vibration that can transform our raw emotion into wisdom, kindness, and compassion. As such, it also holds the power to balance all of the other chakras. Vedic teachings emphasize the role of unconditional love as a necessary quality to achieve the higher spiritual knowledge of Brahman, so it is through opening this chakra that we connect to the infinite divine energy. When this chakra is closed, however, we can experience anger, jealousy, fear of intimacy, and self-loathing. A blocked heart chakra is also linked to cardiopulmonary ailments ranging from asthma to heart disease.

THE FIFTH CHAKRA
THE THROAT CHAKRA (VISHUDDHA)

The throat chakra is located, not surprisingly, in the throat, and is considered the link between the heart and mind; it is related to the ether/Akash element and the anandamaya kosha (the bliss sheath). This energy center represents our connection to truth in that it allows us to communicate and express the emotions, thoughts, and feelings of the other chakras through words; what we think and talk about becomes what we manifest through the power of connection between this chakra and the silent vibrational energy field of Akash, or the zero point field. As such, this chakra is the foundation of the

Vedic reverence for sound: If we are able to open the throat chakra, and deliberately express ourselves both audibly (with words and mantras) and inaudibly (with thoughts and silent mantra meditation), we are able to collaborate with the universal energy field. Put succinctly, it is through sound and the throat chakra that we manifest reality in our lives. A blockage in this chakra can manifest in difficulty expressing feelings, thyroid disease, or physical symptoms such as a frequent sore throat, ear infections, and jaw pain (TMJ).

THE SIXTH CHAKRA
THE THIRD EYE CHAKRA (AJNA)

The third eye chakra is the first of the spiritual chakras. As such, it is not specifically associated with an element or sheath. Located in the center of the forehead, this chakra is the source of intuition and self-knowledge. It controls the endocrine system through the pituitary gland, the tiny pea-shaped organ at the base of the brain that produces many important hormones such as growth hormone and oxytocin. The activation of this chakra is dependent on the sequential opening of all the chakras beneath it, and it is essential to the cultivation of deep states of meditation and a sense of oneness. It also leads to a transcendent mastery of the senses—this is sometimes expressed by people being able to sense future occurrences or being able to read with their eyes closed. There is in fact a well-known homeopathic doctor in Vellore who is able to see with her eyes closed—indeed I've seen her read while blindfolded—because, as she explains it, her third eye chakra has been activated. I myself underwent a traditional initiation with Amma—occurring oftentimes between a student and spiritual teacher—in opening this chakra, in which kumkum, a mixture made of turmeric powder and lemon juice that has been allowed to dry, is applied on the center of the forehead.

THE SEVENTH CHAKRA
THE CROWN CHAKRA (SAHASRARA)

The crown chakra is located on the top of the head. It is the foundation of our spirituality, the center for deeper connection both within ourselves and with Brahman, the source of all creation. When the crown chakra is in balance, we experience a state of universal consciousness, producing a sublime self-awareness as well as an unprejudiced view of the world. This chakra also oversees all the functions of the central nervous system. When this chakra is out of balance, people may experience insomnia and other sleep disturbances, nerve pain, or migraines, as well as difficulty concentrating. Additionally, the crown chakra is linked to the pineal gland, which sends hormonal and electrical messages throughout the body—similar to the way the chakras serve as the channels for subtle energy throughout the body.[8] The pineal gland may also be the physiological juncture where the mind-body connection meets the subtle energy body. Accordingly, when this chakra is opened we have experiences that transcend the five senses entirely. It's not, however, until all the other chakras have been opened that the crown chakra can activate. Individuals who have opened this chakra experience bliss and peace—and a sense of unity within the world—despite tumultuous external circumstances. When the animated life force leaves our body, it is said to leave through this chakra; this chakra connects us directly to the universal energy field.

In addition to their respective element and sheath associations, each chakra is attached to a one-syllable bija mantra. Each bija mantra is a reflection of the resonant sound of the chakra; when one is chanted, the sound vibrates from the chakra into the nervous system and all of the resonant cells of the body. Similar to the scientists of modern times who have been able to amplify the sound of cells and molecules using advanced technological equipment, the Vedic masters (equipped with nothing other than highly attuned minds) were able to perceive and audibly re-create the sound of the chakras on the subtlest level.

When chanted together, these typically make up the chakra mantra. The chakra mantra that Amma taught me, however, is unique because it combines all of the bija mantras with another mantra—Om Namah Shivaya—that is aimed at creating a connection to the universal consciousness through the five elements that serve as the building blocks for the material world. When the mantras are combined in this way, they create a powerful alchemy for a specific purpose—which, here, is to uniformly move energy through all of the chakras, clearing out obstructions to health while also bringing the body into closer participation with the universal energy field.

THE BIJA MANTRAS:

Root Chakra: LAM

Sacral Chakra: VAM

Solar Plexus Chakra: RAM

Heart Chakra: YAM

Throat Chakra: HAM

Third Eye Chakra: OM

Crown Chakra: OM

AMMA'S CHAKRA MANTRA:

The bija mantras combined with Om Namah Shivaya

Note that the mantras are not always spelled the same way when translated for chanting; they are spelled phonetically to make the sound that will reverberate with vibration when vocalized.

HARI OM

NAM, LAM

MAM, VAM

SIM, RAM

VAM, YAM

YAM, HAM

SHIVA OM

SWAHA

PRACTICE:

Chant this mantra aloud for ten minutes for the first three days, fifteen minutes for the next ten days, and then twenty minutes each day thereafter. Once it becomes familiar, you may chant it silently.

Always chant the mantra in full in order to disseminate energy equally throughout the body. I *do not* recommend chanting a single bija mantra—if, for example, you want only to activate the throat chakra— because this can build up disproportionate heat in one area and cause an imbalance.

For those interested in hearing the version of the chakra mantra that my husband and I recorded, you can find it on my website, www.drkulreetchaudhary.com.

To activate all of the chakras, though, there is another energy besides prana, the life-force energy that the chakra mantra calls on, that must come into play. This is called the kundalini energy. To explain how this energy works, though, requires a bit of backstory about Brahman, according to Vedic cosmology. When the universe was first created, the unified energy of Brahman split into Shiva and Shakti, male and female energies respectively, which were subsequently responsible for creating the universe. This pair became the divine masculine and feminine energies underlying all of creation, and Vedic philosophy posits that we are all made up of a combination of these two energies. This split also created the dual experience of life: the underlying, unseen principle of consciousness (Shiva) and the experience of the seen reality of the natural world (Shakti). A common metaphor used to describe this is that Shiva is the blank screen of consciousness upon which Shakti—all vibrating energy—projects creation. It is the movement of Shakti's energy that ultimately creates the universe. It is from this movement that all vibrations, including sound, arise. Of course, the separation between Shiva and Shakti is an illusion—or, in Vedic terms, maya—and the underlying state of unity in the form of Brahman is what all human beings strive to regain.

To regain that oneness, the energy of the divine feminine, Shakti, must also flow through the chakras through a central nadi called the sushumna[9]—a Sanskrit word meaning "very gracious" or "joyful mind"—that runs down the central axis of the body, through the spine, in order to illuminate the chakras. This divine feminine energy, known as kundalini energy, is often described as a coiled snake in Vedic literature and it rests in its potential energy form in the root chakra. The movement of kundalini energy upward through the spine toward the crown chakra is the ultimate aim of mantra meditation practice because it connects a person to the universal energy field—to Brahman—so directly. When this occurs, the divine feminine energy of Shakti unites with the divine masculine energy of Shiva. This reunion represents a return to oneness and the dissolution of the individual ego. When that state is permanently stabilized, we call it enlightenment: Shiva and Shakti, joined once again, merging back into Brahman.

Kundalini energy becomes activated through developing spiritual practices such as yoga, breathing techniques, the use of Ayurvedic/Siddha herbs, spiritual study, and mantra meditation. By combining the bija mantras of the five elements with Om Namah Shivaya, which strengthens our connection with the universal consciousness, Amma's mantra is a vibratory reunion of Shiva and Shakti that activates this divine feminine energy. Kundalini energy can, however, also be activated more directly by an enlightened spiritual teacher performing certain rituals; this is considered the passive activation of kundalini (as opposed to the former, active practices). It is not possible to enter the passive receiving of kundalini activation until a certain degree of mental, physical, and spiritual preparation has taken place.

I think of myself as having spent the ages of nine to forty-three predominantly engaged with the active path of activating my kundalini energy. Now, here in India, I have entered the passive phase. I believe this began when, after Amma taught me the chakra mantra, she placed the kumkum on my forehead that same night. Though she'd done this with me before, there was something about the combination of these two practices that allowed all of my chakras to temporarily open in a way that they never had before. It was one of the most intense and exquisite experiences of my life. Throughout the night, I wasn't dreaming per se, but I was in an altered state. It was my first brush with enlightenment, and it made me realize that uncovering our true selves offers an unbridled joy that defies description. I *can* tell you that I remember thinking it seemed absurd that this much bliss could take the form of a body. How could such an expansive feeling be contained in anything or belong to anyone?

On my trip to India, when I quit my job and left my family behind for three months, I spent the first month feeling deeply uncertain about the decision I had made and unmoored by my lack of communication with Amma. I began to question what exactly I was doing there. So I was relieved when, finally, she invited me to her house for a visit.

When I arrived, I found Amma sitting on her porch, doodling on a piece of paper. As I got closer, I realized that she had written out a list of bija mantras—what I would later learn was the chakra mantra that Amma would so powerfully teach me to chant—and was now creating little curving lines connecting these mantras together. The drawing was taking the familiar shape of a twisted double ladder. As a physician, I knew immediately what Amma was illustrating, but I didn't understand why.

Amma raised her eyes and asked, "What does this look like, Kulreet?"

You could have shown this picture to a thousand medical school students and they'd all have come to the same conclusion.

"It's a drawing of human DNA," I said.

"Yes," Amma replied.

"Why is it drawn around the mantras?" I asked.

"Life on earth was created using a combination of these vibrations, Kulreet," Amma said. "When there are mutations in human DNA, we can correct them using these same sounds."

It seemed like an extravagant claim at the time—though somehow Amma manages to say things with a clarity and serenity that makes anything seem possible. Still, to my delight, I have since found scientific reason to support this. In 2013, researchers at the Benson-Henry Institute for Mind Body Medicine at Massachusetts General Hospital and Beth

Israel Deaconess Medical Center (BIDMC) gathered twenty-six adults with no prior experience with relaxation techniques and enrolled them in an eight-week relaxation response course.[10] Researchers drew blood from the participants before and after their training; for comparison, a set of blood samples was also taken from twenty-five individuals with four to twenty-five years' experience with a regular relaxation practice—various forms of meditation, yoga, and prayer. All of the blood samples were analyzed to determine the expression of more than 22,000 genes.

The results were compelling: Significant changes occurred in the expression of several important groups of genes between the novice samples—the blood drawn from participants before they'd done any relaxation training at all—and those from both the short-term and long-term sets, with the most notable differences appearing in the long-term practitioners. A systems biology analysis revealed that pathways involved with energy metabolism were upregulated during the relaxation response. Furthermore, pathways controlled by activation of a protein called NF-κB—known to have a prominent role in inflammation, stress, trauma, and cancer—were suppressed after the relaxation response training of all lengths. The expression of genes involved in insulin pathways was also considerably altered. In short, mantra meditation, along with other forms of relaxation techniques, can in fact interact with the body on a genomic basis.

The lead researchers on this study[11]—which was published in the peer-reviewed scientific journal *PLOS One*—note that, since this work was done with healthy participants, they are now collaborating with the Dana-Farber Cancer Institute, Massachusetts General Hospital, and Beth Israel Deaconess Medical Center to study the effect of relaxation training on patients with precursor forms—meaning they don't quite meet the criteria of the disease yet but eventually will—of multiple myeloma, a condition known to involve activation of NF-κB pathways.

More recently, in a 2018 study[12] also published in *PLOS One*, scientists from Kyoto University's Graduate School of Biostudies found that certain genes can actually be suppressed when subjected to audible sound. The researchers placed a variety of human cells into an incubator equipped with a full-range loudspeaker, exposed them to a variety of sounds at different frequencies, and then analyzed them. They found that certain genes known as mechanosensitive genes— particularly those that make up bone or skeletal muscle—were suppressed by up to 40 percent after just a couple of hours of exposure, and that those effects lasted for up to four hours. "Our research has found that audible sound stimulation leads to specific genetic response," noted lead researcher Shige H. Yoshimura. The team is now studying how these genetic changes will impact a cell's function, and thus the body as a whole, given that the current results offer convincing evidence that sound can indeed impact DNA.

The idea that our genes can be altered by factors other than what we inherit—such as our environment and stress and diet—is also the foundation for a rapidly growing field in biology called epigenetics. Epigenetics is the study of heritable changes in gene expression that do not involve alteration to the underlying DNA sequence—meaning that an actual gene is not changed but rather the way it is *expressed* is modified—which in turn affects how cells are altered. When DNA is expressed, it is translated into RNA (ribonucleic acid), which acts as a messenger carrying instructions for controlling the synthesis of proteins. Those instructions are translated into proteins that can switch a gene on or off—this, in turn, determines a number of dramatic outcomes, including whether or not an illness occurs.[13] In fact, only 5 to 10 percent of *all* cancer cases can be attributed to heredity[14]—leaving the remaining 90 to 95 percent explained by environment and lifestyle. Other recent studies in this field have brought forth such wide-ranging revelations as the exposure of pregnant women to environmental pollution could increase the babies' risks of developing asthma[15] (and could be passed on epigenetically through several generations[16]) to the finding that descendants of Holocaust survivors may have a chemical coating on their chromosomes causing some to suffer from higher levels of stress and vulnerability.[17] In other words, our parents'—and even our grandparents' and great-grandparents'—experiences may affect our gene expression. The world of medicine has had to incorporate these findings into its understanding of how to treat patients, broadening the scope of treatment to include environmental and lifestyle factors.

Since the surge of interest in genetic assimilation beginning in the 1990s, many have hailed epigenetics as a pioneering and valuable science. Amma's assertion that mantra meditation can change DNA—and the current scientific studies that back it up—is simply another way of saying that sound is a strong epigenetic modifier. A mantra aimed at balancing all of the chakras, as it turns out, has the same scientific validity for altering the expression of certain genes and correcting mutations that would alter the course of an illness. Once again, Ayurvedic medicine serves as a forerunner to the epigenetic findings of today.

6

AYURVEDIC MEDICINE

The doctor of the future will give no medicine, but will interest his patients in the care of the human frame, in diet and in the cause and prevention of disease.

—THOMAS EDISON

Everybody talks about the genes that they received from their mother and father for this trait or the other, but in reality those genes alone have very little impact on life outcomes. Our biology is way too complicated for that and deals with hundreds of thousands of independent factors. "Genes are absolutely not our fate,"[1] pioneer genomic researcher Craig Venter, known for leading the first-draft sequence of the human genome in 2000 with the National Institutes of Health (NIH),[2] once remarked. "They can give us useful information about the increased risk of a disease, but in most cases they will not determine the actual cause of the disease, or the actual incidence of somebody getting it. Most biology will come from the complex interaction of all the proteins and cells working with environmental factors, not driven directly by the genetic code."[3]

It was a forward-thinking speech, a visionary approach to the human genome and our future health, and yet it unwittingly recalled the ancient Eastern traditions—traditional Chinese medicine and Ayurvedic medicine among them—that similarly maintained that we are in constant genetic communication with our environment. Although epigenetics focuses on the physical body—specifically the way that our genes are turned on and off when altered by external circumstances—Eastern medical philosophy considers the subtle energy body as well, maintaining that it, too, has a profound effect on DNA expression and, by extension, our health. The two branches of knowledge have remarkably analogous views on the effects of lifestyle on genetic expression and, subsequently, cellular modification.

Both Eastern and Western traditions, for example, indicate that genetic inheritance is far-reaching in that a trauma suffered by our ancestors might still play out down the line, affecting not only an individual's children but also their children's children and future generations from there. What modern science now calls an "epigenetic imprint" was known as "ancestral karma" in Vedic medicine.

In fact, when experienced Ayurvedic practitioners take the pulse of their patients, we can often glean the traumas from generations past. I once met with a patient—I'll call her Emma—while running my neurology practice in San Diego who was battling severe digestive issues. Though she had been suffering since childhood and had tried a variety of Western treatments and medicines in addition to natural therapies throughout her life, she was still unable to hold down her food much of the time. She frequently either vomited or suffered from diarrhea after eating a meal. Emma was a tall woman, in her late fifties, with a regal presence that shone through despite her being hunched and emaciated due to her disorder. At five foot seven, she was barely ninety pounds. As soon as I felt Emma's pulse, a picture of starving people came into my mind with another flash of a young boy indicating to me that the memory of whatever this was still held in her DNA. "Which generation in your family went through a famine?" I asked.

She blinked a couple of times and then said that a distant relative on her father's side—she believed it was her great-great-great-grandfather—had lived in southern Ireland during the Great Famine, between the years of 1845 and 1849, during which a million people died, the greatest loss of life in nineteenth-century Europe.[4] Many others, including Emma's great-grandfather, emigrated. From that generation onward, the family, including Emma's mother and grandmother, had suffered what they considered to be hereditary digestive issues.

Interestingly and coincidentally, given Emma's situation, the most significant studies of trans-generational transmission of trauma is based on the Dutch Famine, known to those in German-occupied Netherlands as the Hongerwinter,[5] which occurred near the end of World War II when a German blockade cut off food and fuel shipments from farm towns to the northern parts of the country. More than twenty thousand men, women, and children died.[6] Millions of others suffered but survived—among this population were pregnant women whose children, as studies in the 1980s showed, later grew up to

have higher rates of obesity, diabetes, and mental illness. By the
time this group reached old age, the risks increased, according
to L. H. Lumey, an epidemiologist at Columbia University; the
Hunger Winter cohort (as those who were in utero during the
Dutch Famine are referred to by researchers) died at a higher
rate than people before or afterward.[7] "We found a 10 percent
increase in mortality after sixty-eight years," said Dr. Lumey,
who, along with his colleagues, reviewed the death records of
hundreds of thousands of Dutch people born in the mid-1940s.
Furthermore, when the *grandchildren* of men and women exposed to the famine were studied, they, too, were reported to
have had higher rates of illness.[8]

In my work with Emma, I prescribed herbs and mantra meditation, but I also asked that she address and connect with her ancestral history in a way that I felt would release that trauma from
her body. She was dubious, but also determined to wrest her
life back from this mysterious illness. I started by having Emma
chant a bija mantra (I hadn't yet learned the chakra mantra and
so was not prescribing it at this point) as well as work with a
Reiki practitioner to help her make the connection between her
digestive issues and the fear and loss that her great-grandfather
experienced during the Great Famine. She knew a bit of his story
from family lore—that he had large, pale blue eyes, that he'd
seemed a fairly nervous person but very kind, too—and so she
was able to bring some detail to her imagined sense of her great-
grandfather. In doing this, she began to feel a kind of kinship with
him when she thought about him in her mantra meditations.

In India, in order to address ancestral karma,[9] people perform special ceremonies such as the puja ceremony, a spiritual

ritual often used to honor someone after they die (*puja* is a Sanskrit word that means reverence, homage, adoration, worship[10]); sometimes, too, Indian families make an offering on their ancestors' behalf, such as giving a cow to a poor family. In fact, every year Hindus spend fifteen days in a period of ancestor worship called Pitru Paksha devoted to the remembrance of ancestors, during which they donate food to the hungry and reflect on the contributions of their forefathers. In doing a positive thing, and creating good karma, the idea is that you release some of the negative or troubled karma that has been passed down. In Emma's case, I asked that she do something equivalent to honor her family such as making donations to food banks on behalf of her great-grandfather.

The notion that doing good can have meaningful health outcomes was evidenced by a remarkable 2013 study published in the Proceedings of the National Academy of Sciences of the United States of America, wherein a team of professors from the University of North Carolina at Chapel Hill and the University of California, Los Angeles, showed that acts of genuine goodness can have measurable impacts on our genetic expression and health outcomes. According to their research, the human body is able to perceive when the pursuit of well-being is aimed at a noble purpose and when it is being sought for simple self-gratification, and that different gene regulatory programs are engaged for each. When a more "positive affective experience" (i.e., a noble purpose) is the goal, there is a down-regulation of the CTRA gene profile, associated with cardiovascular, neurodegenerative, and neoplastic diseases, which are conditions that cause tumor growths.

Emma had been living for so long as if she, too, were in a famine, that it took us nearly two years to shift her cellular memory and mind toward a healthier track. But, little by little, with Emma's unyielding determination and her willingness to try things that, at first glance, seemed to have little to do with her digestion, her so-called genetic disorder did resolve itself. When we finished working together, Emma was up to 125 pounds and her body was able to metabolize food regularly. It was, from my perspective, quite a beautiful transformation. I was so pleased, of course, that Emma was feeling better, and looking so healthy, but I also enjoyed watching her psychological growth as she unburdened herself of such long-held subconscious anguish.

Ayurvedic medicine—the word *Ayurveda* is derived from the root *ayus* in Sanskrit,[11] meaning "life" or "longevity" and *veda*, meaning "science" or "sacred knowledge"—can be traced back to India five thousand years ago. A description of this practice is found in ancient Vedic texts such as the *Charaka Samhita* and *Sushruta Samhita*, which offer a richly detailed depiction of the physiology and interrelated systems of the body, the variations in human constitution, as well as the use of herbs and herbal mixtures, in addition to other rituals for achieving and maintaining health. It is a complete system for managing *all* aspects of health including healing disease, increasing longevity, performing surgery with precise instruments of their own making, and addressing ethical dilemmas as well as spiritual development.

Ayurvedic medicine also established the system of koshas— or sheaths—and chakras as part of its understanding of the subtle and physical body. As you'll recall, the five sheaths make up the biofield, or subtle energy body; the chakras are the energy centers that transmit the information from the biofield to the body. There is, however, a third part of this diagnostic system that I have not yet portrayed: the doshas.

As with the sheaths and chakras, Ayurvedic medicine considers the human body also to be made up of the five elements (ether, air, fire, water, and earth), though in the case of the body these elements combine to form three fundamental physical-mental-emotional types, or doshas: vata, pitta, and kapha. Discussion of the doshas can be found as far back as Siddha medicine, so it's likely that this philosophy developed earlier and then was in part adopted by Ayurvedic medicine. Creating balance between the physical, mental, and emotional in each of us requires a dynamic harmony among the five elements in the body as expressed through the doshas. Ultimately, these five elements that exist in the universe also exist within us. Where the sheaths and chakras are energetic, however, the doshas are emblematic of what is happening in the entire biofield. In this way, we can draw another parallel to epigenetics: What geneticists call a phenotype is the observable physical interpretation, or characteristic, for a set of genes in the DNA; in Ayurvedic medicine, the doshas offer the observable physical interpretation, or characteristic, of the entire human biofield. Where a geneticist would say that our DNA offers instructions that our bodies follow, an Ayurvedic practitioner would say the biofield offers instructions that our bodies follow. Ultimately, they are both espousing the same fundamental concept—that the body is an expression of information gathered at a primary level.

Ayurvedic medicine takes this idea one step further, however, in that it uses the doshas—which delineate different body-mind types, each with specific responses to diet, seasons, and the environment and each with its own set of predispositions to illness—to make diagnoses and offer health plans for explicit changes in lifestyle, diet, stress, and environment in order to cultivate the highest potential of health in a person.

Each dosha type is defined as a combination of two of the five elements that constitute the universe and a correlated set of qualities. Vata, for example, is a combination of the lighter elements ether and air; this dosha governs all movement, including blood flow, contraction of the heart, breathing, and communication of cells through nerve impulses. Pitta is a combination of fire and water and represents digestion, metabolism, and transformation, including appetite and endocrine functions. Kapha is a combination of the heavier elements of earth and water and regulates structure and cohesion of the body, including strength, fluid balance, and weight. Although Ayurvedic medicine asserts that each person is made up of all three doshas, there is typically one that is dominant. But, just as life isn't static, people can have a combination of two doshas, with one dosha rising to be more powerful at different points in life. Disease, it is believed, is caused in the body by either an excess or a deficiency of vata, pitta, or kapha, which ultimately causes cellular dysfunction.

At the core of Ayurveda is the belief that, by engaging in a meditation practice and by altering our diet and lifestyle according to the dominant dosha or doshas within us, we can modify our genes and alter disease. As an Ayurvedic practitioner, I don't tell all of my patients to eat a vegan diet or that they should all walk ten thousand steps a day; those prescriptions would not benefit every dosha. Instead, I would suggest to someone with a vata physiology to do gentle yoga, while I may tell someone else with a kapha build to aim for twenty thousand steps a day. Ayurvedic medicine also offers behavioral recommendations to improve the mental health or life circumstances for a particular constitution. Again, I would not give the same advice to everyone. A patient who is having trouble with budgeting—be it with time and energy or, speaking more literally, with money—will need different counsel based on the dominant dosha. A vata patient, for instance, is more likely to give far too much away in all circumstances, and therefore I would advise that person on how not to spend down so many resources, financial or otherwise. On the other hand, kapha individuals are more likely to be overly cautious, depleting themselves in a counterintuitive way by spending much of their time and attention on hoarding their energies and coffers. I would encourage this person to behave a bit more freely, offering more of themselves in relationships and making charitable donations. In this way, the doshas offer not only detailed epigenetic prescriptions but a holistic approach to health.

Before we go any further, it will be helpful to know, in a general way, which of the three doshas is commanding your character and constitution. Despite the fact that each of us is, of course, a unique combination of the doshas, best evaluated in person by an Ayurvedic practitioner, the following questions will help you get a basic sense of which one most represents your body and mind.

WHAT IS YOUR DOMINANT DOSHA?

To get a sense of your dominant dosha, answer the questions below:

FRAME

a) I am thin and slender with prominent joints and lean muscles.

b) I have a medium, symmetrical build with good muscle development.

c) I have a large or stocky build.

SKIN

a) My skin is dry and rough.

b) My skin is warm, reddish in color, and easily irritated.

c) My skin is moist and oily.

HAIR

a) My hair is dry, brittle, or frizzy.

b) My hair is fine, thin, or prematurely gray.

c) My hair is thick and wavy.

EYES

a) My eyes are small and active.

b) I have a penetrating gaze.

c) I have large pleasant eyes.

JOINTS

a) My joints are thin, prominent, and have a tendency to crack.

b) My joints are loose and flexible.

c) My joints are large, well knit, and firm.

BODY TEMPERATURE

a) My hands and feet are usually cold and I prefer warm environments.

b) I am usually warm, regardless of the season, and prefer cooler environments.

c) I am adaptable to most temperatures but do not like cold, wet days.

UNDER STRESS . . .

a) I become anxious or worried.

b) I become irritable, intense, or aggressive.

c) I become withdrawn or depressed.

SLEEP

a) I am a light sleeper with a tendency to awaken easily.

b) I am a moderately sound sleeper, usually needing less than eight hours to feel rested but have vivid dreams.

c) My sleep is deep and long. I tend to awaken slowly in the morning.

WEATHER

a) My least favorite is cold weather.

b) My least favorite is hot weather.

c) My least favorite is damp weather.

WEIGHT

a) I tend to lose weight easily.

b) I maintain my weight easily.

c) I gain weight easily.

APPETITE

a) On a daily basis, my appetite varies and I have delicate digestion.

b) I feel uncomfortable if I skip a meal and I can eat almost anything.

c) I like to eat, but can skip meals easily. I have a slow digestion.

BOWEL MOVEMENTS

a) Tend to be hard with occasional constipation.

b) Tend to be loose with occasional diarrhea.

c) Tend to be well-formed or sticky with occasional constipation.

PERSONALITY

a) I am lively and enthusiastic by nature. I like change.

b) I am purposeful and intense. I like being efficient and in control.

c) I am easygoing and caring. I like to support others.

ACTIVITY

a) I like to be active, and it can be hard to sit still.

b) I enjoy activity that has a purpose, especially competitive.

c) I like leisurely activities and staying home.

WALK

a) I walk quickly.

b) I have a determined walk.

c) I walk slowly and steadily at a leisurely pace.

MOODS

a) My moods change quickly, with a tendency toward anxiety.

b) My moods change slowly, but I can become angry easily.

c) My moods are mostly steady and most things don't bother me.

MEMORY

a) I learn quickly and forget quickly.

b) I have a good memory.

c) I learn slowly but have a good long-term memory.

ORGANIZATION

a) I am good at getting things started, but not at getting things done.

b) I am very organized and can focus on a project from start to finish.

c) I need help getting things started, but I am good at seeing things to the finish.

MONEY

a) I spend money almost as quickly as I make it.

b) It is important for me to have money and I spend it on expensive, luxury items.

c) I don't like to spend money and prefer saving it for a rainy day.

IN RELATIONSHIPS I USUALLY ASK . . .

a) What is wrong with me?

b) What is wrong with you?

c) Are you sure there is something wrong?

OUT OF BALANCE, I FEEL LIKE . . .

a) A leaf in the wind.

b) A raging inferno.

c) A bump on a log.

MY MOTTO IN LIFE IS . . .

a)   Throw caution to the wind and live for today.

b)   No pain no gain.

c)   Don't worry, be happy.

If you chose mostly A's: You are primarily vata.

If you chose mostly B's: You are primarily pitta.

If you chose mostly C's: You are primarily kapha.

The Ayurvedic plan offered for each dosha has thorough instructions for daily and seasonal routines—including the time to go to bed and when to wake up, the time to eat, the time to exercise, and the time to meditate, among other activities. Diet and nutrition are advised right down to the texture and qualities of the food; the season and even geographic location of the person are considered when tailoring a diet for each dosha. It also has recommendations for proper behavior, and how to deal with peers, as well as those who are younger and older. Broadly, advice and guidance should be given to those who are younger, for example, and respect should be given to teachers and elders. Love and compassion should be extended above all else. These behaviors, Ayurvedic medicine signifies, affect health on the physical level so it is not just to make the world a better place—it also happens to restore the mind and body.

It should not surprise you that in addition to these recommendations, each dosha has a specific bija mantra meant to bring the body back into balance. Typically, it is recommended to chant the bija mantra for at least fifteen minutes a day once the dosha imbalance has been identified. Start by chanting out loud and then, once it feels comfortable to do so, chant it silently in your mind. Continue to chant this mantra in your practice until the symptoms of dosha imbalance resolve. (For example, this will be apparent when the qualities of a vata dosha feel more grounded or those of a pitta dosha feel cooled down or when someone who has balanced a kapha dosha feels more stimulated.) Once this occurs, revert to the chakra mantra, which is great for keeping all of the doshas in maintenance. The bija mantras for the doshas are a correction for an acute issue in the short term, whereas the chakra mantra is a form of long-term maintenance.

VATA

A person with predominant vata tends to be slight and fine-boned; Audrey Hepburn was a good example of this type. Vata represents movement, as I mentioned, for all bodily processes; its characteristics are dry, light, quick, cold, rough, subtle, mobile, and clear. On a seasonal basis, vata is at its peak in the fall, when it is generally windy and dry at the change of seasons. Vata types are always in motion—they are alert and tend to walk and talk fast; they grasp concepts quickly but also forget them just as quickly; and they are flexible in their ideas and creativity. As such, one of the basic principles for this dosha is to create regularity in the daily routine to help ground the moving energy.

In the body, vata resides in the colon, brain, ears, bones, joints, skin, and thighs. Vata people tend to be more susceptible to diseases involving the principle of air—such as emphysema and pneumonia—as well as arthritis, gas, dry skin and hair, neurological conditions, constipation, and mental confusion.

When out of balance, vata individuals can feel unstable in the midst of change; they also become fearful, nervous, and anxious. Given their wiry energy, vata types fatigue easily and often need a lot of sleep.

The bija mantras prescribed to help bring vata back into balance are those that help calm the hyperactive qualities of this dosha. The first is Hrim (pronounced *hreem*), which is a specific mantra for the heart, emphasizing the physical health of the heart but also creativity and compassion. The second is Klim (pronounced *kleem*), which promotes blood flow and digestion as well as smooth skin. It can also help calm the brain and boost the reproductive and immune systems.

PITTA

Pitta individuals exemplify many of the qualities of fire: hot, intense, penetrating, sharp, and agitated. As such, pittas are high achievers, ambitious and driven: think Steve Jobs. Success, accomplishment, and satisfaction in one's activity are important for pitta individuals.

Pitta is dominant, appropriately given the blazing nature of this dosha, during the summer. The tendency of pitta is to get overheated and impatient; the basic principle, therefore, for keeping pitta in balance is to keep it cool—physically and emotionally.

Two cooling bija mantras that are useful for balancing this

dosha are: Aim (pronounced *aym*), which opens the voice and lungs and clears the senses, and Srim (pronounced *shreem*), which can boost overall energy and concentration as well as feelings of nurturance.

KAPHA

The qualities of kapha are heavy, steady, slow, cold, soft, and solid. Kapha individuals, consequently, tend to have a slow metabolism, shun exercise, and gain weight easily. They have large physical frames but with well-developed muscles and joints. Physically, kaphas have a great deal of strength, stamina, and endurance. They learn slowly but their long-term memory is excellent. They tend to be deep sleepers and often have trouble waking up in the morning.

When kapha types are in balance, they tend to be generous, have loving personalities, and remain stable and grounded in the midst of chaos—they are like the eye of a hurricane. Oprah Winfrey strikes me as a kapha in this way. When kapha individuals get out of balance, however, they can experience greed, possessiveness, and lethargy. The key to keeping kapha in balance is to stay mentally and physically stimulated.

Kapha individuals are more likely to have disease connected to the water principle such as flu, sinus congestion, excess mucus production, obesity, diabetes, water retention, and headaches. Winter and spring are the seasons when kapha accumulates most in the body, and spring is an ideal time for seasonal detoxification programs because kapha begins to "thaw" as the temperature gets warmer, and toxins are ready to be released from the body.

There are two warm and stimulating bija mantras that help to balance the kapha dosha. Hum (pronounced *hoom*) stimulates energy throughout the body from the digestive tract to the immune system to the brain. Dum (pronounced *doom*) is, despite its phonetic spelling, intended to create protective energy, spiritually and physically.

The healing power of mantras and sound is inextricably woven into Ayurvedic medicine. Mantras are a vehicle for raising individual consciousness to universal consciousness while also reversing both mental and physical disorders. Bija mantras are a potent way to alter the body, and a crucial part of the prescription, then, when helping a patient to balance the koshas—or the biofield—as well as the doshas.

Just as important, mantras also once played a fundamental role in the preparation of medicine. Traditionally, the entire process was, in fact, inseparable from sound. In order to train to be an Ayurvedic doctor, the student would first live with his teacher and engage in a committed mantra practice meant to enliven the consciousness of the aspiring Ayurvedic physician. When the guru deemed his student to be receptive enough to receive the knowledge of Ayurvedic medicine, he would begin to plant the seeds for the Ayurvedic herbs—chanting a specific mantra for each one. When the herbs were harvested, again another mantra was engaged; these mantras were chanted yet again while the herbs were administered to patients.

Over the last several hundred years, however, as Ayurvedic

medicine has become more popular and institutionalized in India, it has been taught in a method akin to Western medicine. Sadly, modern life does not allow for the kind of undertaking that training to be an Ayurvedic practitioner once required; there are only a few people left in the world who were taught in the classic way.

Thanks to my childhood mantra practice, I have inadvertently approached the study of Ayurveda in the traditional way, and because of this early exposure to mantra meditation, its profound influence in Ayurveda was a natural connection for me to make as I shifted my neurology practice toward integrative medicine. Most modern-day Ayurvedic physicians, however, have not been raised with a mantra meditation practice and therefore don't have a full appreciation for how important a role it plays in this system. Over time, the discipline as a whole has become less holistic and, in general, the mantra is no longer used during the preparation of the herbs—they are made in factories. Ironically enough, many modern Ayurvedic physicians focus mainly on physical complaints, dismissing mental and spiritual complaints as irrelevant to the practice of Ayurveda. Sadly, without the ability to purify and equip the mind of the healer with a mantra practice as well as strengthen the effect of the herbs—and without a mantra practice as part of the prescription for patients—the benefit is not nearly as effective. Psychological conditions, in particular, are much more difficult to cure through herbs and diet alone.

Returning to the ancient traditions of sound in Ayurvedic medicine is essential to the efficacy of this discipline. Without it, it is impossible to understand the full nature of the human body or its ultimate goal of attaining access to the higher consciousness, and energy, of Brahman. To that end, we must turn to the earliest notions of sound within Ayurvedic medicine and explore the ancient philosophy of yoga.

7

THE YOGA OF SOUND

Yoga is like music: the rhythm of the body, the melody of the mind,
and the harmony of the soul create the symphony of life.

—B. K. S. IYENGAR

Yoga was not always about flexibility and a good workout. It
wasn't even always a system of physical movements. In the
beginning, yoga was simply a word—albeit a compelling one.
Meaning "union" in Sanskrit, yoga embodied the nearly timeless concept of a human being encountering the Divine. It
was this sense of communing with something larger—call it
Brahman, God, or the energy underlying all being—that Vedic philosophers and Siddha masters held in mind when they
developed the intricate understanding of the human biofield,
with its sheaths, chakras, and doshas. These medical systems,
of course, offered ways in which to balance the body and
mind, and maintain health, but the ultimate aim of Ayurvedic
and Siddha medicine was to help a person open to a universal
energy. Merging back into infinite consciousness was an idea

infused in the Vedas and Siddha records; it was woven into the hymns and poems and mythologized in stories. Yoga, in the original sense of the word, recognizes that emotions are vital and sacred and can offer access, when a person is able to tap into the vibrational universe, to a healthy and meaningful life.

The first mention of yoga is in one of the oldest surviving texts of any Indo-European language: the Rigveda.[1] Historians and linguistic experts speculate that the earliest parts of this collection of Vedic Sanskrit hymns, philosophical questions, and commentaries on liturgy, ritual, and mysticism were written in 1500 to 1200 BC.[2] Over time, the concept of yoga was refined by the Vedic priests as well as the mystic seers known as rishis; they detailed their practices and beliefs in the Upanishads, which offer many of the central philosophical ideas and concepts of Hinduism. The influential German philosopher Arthur Schopenhauer, upon reading the Upanishads, translated into English in the nineteenth century, declared that they were "the production of the highest human wisdom."[3] Among the most well known of the yogic scriptures is the Bhagavad-Gîtâ (scholars debate the date it was written, placing it anywhere between the fifth and second centuries BC), which describes four main yogic paths to realize meaning in life and reach enlightenment. These paths, all of which teach us to surrender the ego, are the yoga of action and service (karma), knowledge (jnana), devotion (bhakti), and self-discipline (raja). "Yoga," as it is described in the Bhagavad-Gîtâ, "is the journey of the Self, through the Self, to the Self."

Vedic philosophy posits that through a dedicated practice of any one of these four paths, a person can achieve self-realization—

the ability to fully accept oneself and others as well as life's circumstances—and attain yoga. It's emblematic of the yogic affability that there are four passages to enlightenment to choose from—this is meant to accommodate the differences in people's natures.

Karma yoga is the path of selfless action, counseling its spiritual seekers to pursue liberation through service and work for the benefit of others.[4] The word *karma* translates from Sanskrit as "to act"; as such, karma yoga considers the cause and effect of human action. Offering one's services or making contributions are ways not only of creating good karma but also of negating any bad karma of the past. These offerings must be authentic—if a person performs a kindness with a hidden wish to gain something in return, the act is not fulfilling its highest purpose. Yet karma yoga also acknowledges that it is natural for people to want something in return for their efforts. Through altruistic service to others, practitioners of karma yoga hope to become keenly aware of their ego and to consistently coax themselves away from self-interest.

This kind of generosity is a key aspect of many Eastern religions: In Buddhism, members of society offer food to monks as an act of selfless service. In Islam, it is expected that Muslims donate to charity. In Sikhism, every temple provides food to anyone who enters. In Hindu mythology, the deities are illustrated as being in service to humanity without any expectations in return. Karma yoga is, in the apt description given by Stan van Hooft in *The Handbook of Virtue Ethics*, "ethically fine-tuned action."[5] This is also inherent, incidentally, in the Hindu ritual of Pitru Paksha, the annual fifteen-day ancestor-worship period I mentioned in the previous chapter, during which people make contributions—such as donating food—on behalf of their relatives.

Jnana yoga, or the yoga of knowledge, requires a constant self-inquiry and uncompromising investigation into the true nature of reality in order to transcend identification with thoughts and ego. In contrast to karma yoga, this is an intense inward practice, involving meditation and philosophical reflection. In the Bhagavad-Gîtâ, it is described as the most difficult and complex approach, as it deals with "formless reality"; it is the yoga that the intellectually ambitious tend to choose. The ultimate goal of jnana yoga is atma jnana, or the realization of the true Self. When this realization dawns, the boundaries of the ego dissolve and the jnana practitioner experiences both infinite wisdom and unconditional love. It has occurred to me, in my study of quantum physics, that these pioneering scientists are somewhat like modern-day jnana yogis in their dogged explorations of the underlying nature of the universe, bringing them into a deeper understanding of the unity of all life.

Bhakti yoga involves a loving commitment to a personal god, making this the most accessible path, since everyone—young or old, rich or poor, healthy or sick, educated or unlearned—can practice devotion. A bhakti yogi is always searching for and honoring the thread of love that connects all of creation. Their constant search for the unity creates an intellectual and emotional awareness that life is in fact just an expression of one underlying reality. This encourages a person to shift the attention from the desires of the individual ego to the intelligence of universal consciousness. It also emphasizes feeling and emotion,

recognizing that the discerning qualities of the intellect are de-
fenseless in the face of tragedy or illness. A bhakti yogi accepts
the challenges of life rather than analyzing or imposing a sense
of control over the circumstances; surrender to divine will is
an essential element of this practice. The bhakti practitioner
cultivates a confidence that everything needed for his or her
spiritual maturation and material well-being will be provided,
trusting that knowledge and wisdom will eventually come. A
feeling of devotion shifts the attention from the desires of the
individual ego—and the external—to the compassion and intelligence of the universal consciousness and the divine within.

Once Amma, while giving a lecture on bhakti yoga—the
branch of yoga that she is a guru within—illustrated her sense
of what it means to trust that there is the divine within us. "If
someone asks, 'Can you show divine?' it is not possible," she
said. "Because divine is not far away from you. Divine is within
you. If something is here"—and she put her hand out at arm's
length—"At this distance, are we able to read? When it comes
here"—she moved her hand closer—"Are we able to read?" She
moved her hand once more so that it was almost touching her face.
"Here?" And then, smiling, she put her hand on her face. "Here?"
Her audience laughed. "That's why we can't see divine. So who
can help us to see it when it is this close? Unless we prepare, unless we are ready, no one can help us to see [the divine]."

Importantly, of the four yogic paths, bhakti yoga is the most
closely connected to sound. The tradition of kirtan, or devo-
tional singing, and mantra—one of the most direct and effective practices for quieting the mind—grew out of bhakti yoga
as essential tools for cultivating devotion.

Raja yoga, associated with self-control, or in its literal translation "the king of the yogas,"[6] is the fourth path. This is often
referred to as classical yoga and was added in more modern clas-
sifications; its origins are unclear.[7] It is known, however, that
the practice was first popularized by the book *Yoga Sutras of
Patanjali*, a collection of aphorisms about the theory and practice of yoga compiled by the sage Patanjali, estimated by some
historians to have been published in 400 BC.[8] Patanjali was
himself a Siddha, one of the many who shared their knowledge
and expertise, hoping to offer it outside of their direct lineage.
The *Yoga Sutras* synthesized many of the Indian philosophical
systems and later became the most translated ancient Indian text
in the medieval era. Raja yoga offered a way to harness the
thoughts of the mind through, Patanjali instructed, a combination of a scrupulous moral and behavioral code—optimism for
oneself, the acceptance of others, and perseverance are among
the many criteria—and a disciplined mantra meditation practiced while holding a still posture and controlling the breath.[9]
The ultimate aim was to achieve samadhi, a state in which the
meditator becomes so absorbed that he or she loses a sense of
identity. Samadhi has also been described as collapsing the three
categories of consciousness: witness, witnessing, and witnessed
(foreshadowing the quantum physics observer effect); it is a sense
of pure consciousness, or oneness—it *is* yoga, the union with
Brahman or the indivisible Self. To obtain this yoga, just as a
king exercises control over his kingdom, so, too, must the practitioner over his mind. Raja yoga, or classical yoga, is the oldest
system of yoga to be developed into a unified practice, bringing
together philosophical aspects with both posture and breathing.

Beginning in the twelfth century BC, Patanjali's text fell into obscurity. It wasn't until seven centuries later, in the late nineteenth century, that Swami Vivekananda, a Hindu monk, helped the book to gain prominence again when he adapted many of Patanjali's ideas into his own version of Hindu religiosity, about which he lectured extensively in the West. In 1896, he published his own book, *Raja Yoga*.[10] It became an instant success and was highly influential in shaping the Western understanding of yoga. In *Raja Yoga*, Vivekananda offered the four paths of yoga, as I've just explained them, as well as an early form of hatha, a branch of yoga that had emerged in the eleventh century, though he did not explicitly call it this. Later, one of his disciples, Swami Abhedananda, taught Americans hatha yoga, including the asanas (postures or, literally, "manner of sitting" in Sanskrit) such as the lotus pose.[11] From here, the yoga as most of us know it today began to take form, blending Western styles of gymnastics with postures from hatha yoga throughout the twentieth century, eventually becoming so popular that it all but obliterated the original meaning of the word and its meditative and sacred core.

And yet, despite the fact that these timeless philosophies are not referred to as yoga within different faiths, the underlying themes are easily perceived: service (karma), knowledge (jnana), devotion (bhakti), and self-discipline (raja).

The concept of yoga in its full and ancient meaning did, however, eventually make its way into Western culture, under the cover of a new theory, thanks to Swiss psychiatrist Carl Jung, who, along with his onetime mentor Sigmund Freud, shaped the modern psychoanalytic movement.[12] Though there is a history, prior to Jung, of Western scholars bringing tenets of Eastern philosophy into their work—Schopenhauer being one of the first—Jung was a pioneer in championing these ideas within a psychological framework. Both Jung and Freud focused on the personal subconscious—comprised of the emotions, wishes, and memories we have forgotten or repressed—but Jung went one step further, suggesting that there is also a *collective* unconscious. This shared information, as he explained it, is comprised of ancestral memory and experience and it exists in everyone. Jung believed that this deeper stratum of the human mind was made up of archetypes, images, and events—such as the apocalypse, the trickster, and death, respectively. These archetypes are inherited potentials made uniquely manifest in each of us.[13] "[Archetypes] only acquire solidity, influence, and eventual consciousness in the encounter with empirical facts, which touch the unconscious aptitude and quicken it to life," Jung wrote. "They are, in a sense, the deposits of all our ancestral experiences, but they are not the experiences themselves."[14] Given Jung's fascination and familiarity with Eastern philosophy, it is not far-fetched to point out the likeness between the collective unconscious—a psychic soup of shared memory—and the Akash, a field believed to record every human event, thought, and emotion.

Jung believed that the thoughts and behaviors we find intolerable are banished to the unconscious and, there, become a "shadow." Everyone carries such a shadow, Jung theorized, and the less it is embodied in a person's conscious life, the blacker and denser it becomes. In order to achieve psychological coherence, a person goes through the process of individuation, which surfaces in both the personal and collective unconscious, integrating them into the conscious mind.[15] Only then can a person experience a genuine realization of the Self; only then can a person achieve the "totality of the whole psyche," as Jung put it.[16]

This process of individuation can be likened to jnana yoga in its intellectual and methodical pursuit of awareness—Jung's individuation process was similarly introspective, stripping away the self to uncover repressed memories (i.e., the shadow), and entering into a "long process of negotiation" with an ultimate aim of opening oneself.[17] "Eastern yoga is based upon man as he really is," Jung once wrote in a letter to a would-be patient, "but we have a conscious imagination about ourselves and think this is our Self, which is an appalling mistake."[18] This individuation process, the integration of the shadow into the Self, is, as with jnana yoga, a long and arduous process and is not guaranteed to happen, even with a committed effort, in a person's lifetime.

Jung also believed that there was a counterpart to our darker unconscious selves—what is sometimes referred to as "the golden shadow"[19]—that contained a more positive potential. We also hide away parts of ourselves, Jung suggested, that are so magnificent and powerful that we struggle to take conscious ownership of them. Again, it is easy to compare Jung's theory to Vedic philosophy: as you will recall, maya is the illusion we cling to because we are too afraid to imagine how we exist as Brahman, without identity or boundary. The "golden shadow" comprises our most creative and noble qualities; this offers a capacity beyond measure and reunites us with our true natures. To connect with and transcend our shadow selves is to achieve union.[20]

Jung felt that the best practice to achieve total integration of the Self was psychoanalysis. The Eastern approach to discovering one's true Self, the divine force, requires cultivating stillness and openness in order to merge with the universal energy of Brahman. And, in the Vedic view, one of the most effective ways to cultivate this state is through a combination of devotion and sound—chanting, music, and mantra.

Nāda yoga is a Vedic practice entirely devoted to sound. The Sanskrit word *nāda* literally means "sound," and yoga, as you now well know, means "union"; nāda yoga, then, is "union through sound." Nāda yogis believe that sound vibrations—rather than matter and particles—are what comprise the universe. This was not only a philosophical structure but also a form of medicine; nāda yoga is the prototype for sound medicine as we know it today. Nāda practitioners, therefore, used sound—engaging mantras and chanting and classical Indian instruments—to create vibrations and resonance within their patients to regulate the immune system as well as treat physical ailments and psychological difficulties. Believing that sound could communicate more than was possible to discern from sensory perceptions and commonplace language alone, they felt that cosmic sound could achieve a more direct and profound unity between ourselves and Brahman, or universal energy.

There are four levels of sound in nāda yoga: Vaikhari, Madhyama, Pashyanti, and Para Nāda. Vaikhari are sounds that are audible to us, such as speech and song. Madhyama—which means "in the middle" in Sanskrit—is a subtler sound, such as a whisper. Pashyanti are mental sounds, like a song that cycles through your mind, the words in a dream, or a silently chanted mantra. Para Nāda cannot be perceived by the human ear and is beyond speech, considered to exist in another dimension; the result is pure silence—or transcendence. It is believed that within this level of transcendental sound is the state in which the Siddhas were able to perceive the mantras they then passed on through oral history to the world.

More broadly, the nāda yoga system divides sounds into two categories: internal, or anahata, and external, or ahata. Ahata sounds are the struck sounds. Like Vaikhari, these are sounds we can perceive through our ears when vibrations are transmitted through our ossicles to the sensory receptors of our inner ears. Conversely, anahata sounds are the unstruck sounds, the individual vibrations of one's own being. Nāda practitioners believe that the anahata—which is a form of Para Nāda—is so closely associated with one's Self that it cannot be physically shared with anyone else. This inner sound, the internal music we each carry, can be heard only by achieving ultimate stillness and quietness, as one can through mantra meditation. When the mind becomes absorbed in one's own anahata sound, it no longer listens so much as resonates, vibrating in unison with it until oneness with Brahman is achieved.[21]

The use of music and sounds to connect to a higher state of consciousness was, and still is, a common practice in a variety of Hindu spiritual traditions as well as other ancient cultures. It has been reported that the Himba tribe in Africa, for instance, believes that a mother can hear the unique song of her baby even before conception. On the day that a woman believes that she will become a mother, she is asked to sit quietly and listen for the song of her baby. When she hears it, she returns to the father and teaches it to him. When they try to conceive, they sing that child's song to invite him or her into the world. Once pregnant, the mother teaches the child's song to the midwives and other women of the village. At birth, the women sing the song to welcome the baby into the world.

As the child matures, more members of the community are taught the child's song. If the child is hurt, someone will sing the song. If the child does something of merit, the village sings this song as a form of honor and acknowledgment. If the child commits a crime, the village will once again gather around to sing, offering community rather than punishment. The birth song is continually and periodically sung throughout the child's life. It's sung to celebrate marriages and other rites of passage. When the child is dying, the tribe sings the song for the last time.

The rites of the Himba tribe also illustrates a powerful and essential element in the bhakti and nāda yoga traditions: the emotional component of a mantra practice is critical for the mantra to have an impact. A mantra, according to the bhakti yoga tradition, cannot be chanted in a perfunctory manner—there must be a feeling of love or devotion to enliven it.

The Vedic masters and Siddhas knew intuitively that emotions play a critical role not just in the mind but also in the body. Not surprisingly, modern medicine has been slower to recognize the physiological impact of emotion. In the early

2000s, as part of my training as a neurologist, I was taught that emotions originated in the brain, which was the prevailing neurological theory at that time. These days, however, the medical community has begun to recognize that emotions are more accurately described as a product of the brain and body acting in concert. As we have seen, research on HRV suggests that we can initially experience emotions physiologically and not just cognitively. The variation in heart rate influences our brains through a shift in neurochemistry, indicating that the heart plays a crucial role in informing our emotional experience. Interestingly, this research parallels the Vedic understanding of the heart chakra as the emotional center of the biofield. In Ayurveda, too, there is an aspect, or subdosha, of pitta known as sadhaka pitta that is believed to connect the heart and brain through the processing of emotions. Interestingly, bringing us full circle, sadhaka pitta is also believed to transform sound into nerve impulses in the brain. The link between sound, emotion, heart, and mind has been confirmed by modern science. Neuroscientific research has found[22] that listening to music causes the release of the neurotransmitter dopamine, an essential signaling molecule that transmits pleasure. From both ancient and modern medical perspectives, then, it is clear that emotion and sound—particularly mantra and music—are capable of affecting the heart and mind, potentially allowing us to move beyond the ego-bound self in a transformative way.

The aim of an integrative practice—and of Ayurvedic medicine—ultimately goes beyond the body. In my practice,

I had often seen patients resolve their physical issues, only to find that they were still left with difficult questions. "What impact am I having on my family?" some would ask, for instance, once they had the distance and energy to see that their illness may have had—may still be having—a reverberating effect. "How am I participating in my community?" others would ask. "What is the purpose of life?" the brave ones would say. That is, once the body is in balance, it is important that I keep working with my patients to bring their spiritual concerns to the conscious mind in order for them to explore a yogic path.

For example, I once had a patient—I'll call him Tim—who came to see me while I was at Scripps. He was a painter with a thriving career; he had a committed, decades-old marriage and two wonderful children. He also had multiple sclerosis. When he came to see me, he was struggling with the physical symptoms of this illness—his right leg was weak on one side, making it difficult for him to walk without a noticeable limp. Just as important, he suffered severe bouts of depression.

In the time that Tim and I worked together he was an ideal patient: He was enthusiastic, exercised regularly, ate healthily, and he took his medications routinely. We worked in a traditional integrative way, helping him incorporate more of an Ayurvedic diet into his life, as well as herbs and yoga asanas. I asked him to take part in a purification therapy called panchakarma—a personalized process that involves various treatments such as massage, herbal enemas, and steam therapy, among other things, to help eliminate toxins and strengthen the immune system; I also put him on an antidepressant that he later tapered off. After two years, Tim was immensely improved. He no longer felt physical limitations due to his MS and his depression was under control. Tim was thrilled about this change in circumstances and I was, of course, thrilled for him.

A few months later, however, Tim came back to see me: He had begun to feel flat in an indistinct, existential way and wondered if there was something we could do. From the perspective of a Western doctor, there was nothing else to do. He was in optimum health—remarkably, he was in better athletic shape than I was after two years of Ayurvedic interventions! But, from an Eastern viewpoint, this dullness was a significant symptom. Tim had, in the parlance of the Vedics, improved his physical sheath, the annamaya sheath, significantly, bringing him closer to his core sheaths—manomaya, the mind sheath, vijñānāmāyā, the wisdom sheath, and anandamaya, the bliss sheath—all of which closely surround the vast universal energy that influences our lives. I felt that if I could bring Tim in closer contact to the energy held within these core sheaths— what Jung might call the subconscious programming of his ego—he would begin to have more insight into the existential sluggishness he was experiencing.

Tim had been to therapy for most of his adult life to explore the significant physical abuse he suffered within his family as a child—the catalyst for his periodic bouts of depression. But he told me that what he was struggling with at this point was a separate emotional difficulty because many of the other symptoms associated with his past episodes of depression were absent.

I asked him if he would be willing to try a mantra practice.

He was, as usual, not just willing but ready to throw himself completely into it—I wouldn't have been surprised if he'd come back the next day having silently meditated for an hour already. I talked to him about the concept of bhakti yoga, explaining that at its core is a feeling of devotion, or unconditional love, that can be helpful in letting go of a constraining sense of identity in order to touch on something more profound. I also explained nāda yoga, in relationship to bhakti yoga, and the use of mantra to alter the body and mind vibrationally.

Finally, I taught him the chakra mantra and asked him if he could think of anything or anyone from his life that inspired a sense of reverence in him. I tend to guide my patients toward something that stirred this feeling in childhood, as I believe this offers a primal emotion, one that is more deeply rooted in them. Some people choose a religious icon, while others name family members. In Tim's case, images of Mother Mary had conveyed a sense of maternal comfort and love to him from a very young age; he'd latched on to these images as a kind of vision of maternal warmth since his own familial circumstances were so dire. I asked him to practice his chakra mantra meditation as a silent ritual—for twenty minutes, once a day at the same time each day, beginning by lighting a candle and looking at a picture of Mother Mary, with the hope that it would invoke a feeling of spiritual connection and unconditional love in him during his practice.

I remember well the day that Tim came in for a visit, about six months into his mantra practice, and explained to me that he felt he'd been blasted open. Tears were streaming down his face—an emotional dam had clearly been torn down. It turned out that a few weeks prior, he had put up a photo of his wife next to the picture of Mary. Throughout his meditations, he had come to feel a deep gratitude—a reverence of its own kind—for his wife and the care with which she had always conducted their relationship. Though she worked full-time and was a committed parent, she was also always present for her husband; she had been particularly supportive since he'd received his MS diagnosis twenty years earlier. She kept him steady in the face of his disease and played a tremendous role in maintaining his health—from helping to adhere to an Ayurvedic diet to making it possible for him to sleep in when he was feeling knocked out by his illness to always remaining steady in the face of a good deal of psychic tumult.

As he talked, the feeling of love he felt for his wife was palpable to me, and I knew that he was cultivating a true bhakti yoga practice. The love that Tim felt for his wife—deep and energizing and sacred—was a reflection of the larger love that animates the divine Self, or the noble and creative shadow in Jung's understanding of individuation. It is the *feeling* of devotion or love or reverence (any one of these is a building block toward a sense of union) then—not rote belief or ritual—that shifts the biology of a person.

Tim was not simply chanting a mantra; he had achieved the sense of union that I hope for on behalf of all of my patients. By infusing his own practice with devotion, he not only opened himself to his wife's love, but also opened toward union with the divine love at the core of his Self. He'd created an authentic yogic practice by enriching the sound of his mantra with positive emotion. This made it possible for him to alter both his heart and mind, liberating him from the constraints of his ego, which held the trauma of childhood, and allowing him to push past the subconscious malaise that had been pervading his life. This is the path of yoga.

8

MANTRA

A person doesn't hear sound only through the ears; he hears sound through every pore of his body. It permeates the entire being.

—SUFI MUSICIAN, HEALER, AND MYSTIC
HAZRAT INAYAT KHAN

"The form of God is energy. The structure of energy is vibration," Amma once expounded in a discourse about mantras. "The cosmic force, or universal force, or what we call God, is just in the form of energy that exists everywhere in creation, including within humans." Most important, this energy, and the vibrations held within it, can be engaged through sound. Throughout history and the world today there are traditions that use distinctive phrases and chants to invoke physical, emotional, and spiritual states: the Gregorian chants of Christianity; the Egyptian use of sound for clearing the chakras; the mystic syllables of the Hebrew alphabet in Kabbala; the Shamanic healers' prayers; Islam's call to prayer; Tibetan Buddhist monks' chants in preparation for meditation. In every one of these traditions exists a vibratory pattern imbued with wisdom and spirituality that can be accessed by sound.

As I detailed earlier in this book, modern science, particularly within the field of quantum physics, has reached a similar conclusion that waveforms—in the form of sound or light—carry an unimaginable quantity of information. (Sound and light are also, of course, all vibrations, but, in science, they are typically referred to as waveforms.) In an earlier scientific understanding, it was believed that space was filled with ether, which, according to Isaac Newton, "could provide a mechanism for gravitational attraction," allowing for the movement of electromagnetic and gravitational forces. A century later, quantum physics revised this view of the subtle material of space and how it might contain and transmit energetic vibrations, offering a vision of the zero point field as the collective ground state energy of space with vibratory patterns held within it, as well as emanating from it.

The Siddhas were among the first to intuit that this universal energy and vibration could be tapped by sound.[1] These were the ancient sages and the rishis, or the mystic seers, who, more than eight thousand years ago, discovered they were able to transcend consciousness, connecting to universal energy, once they were able to train their emotions and minds to stay still. "Who were the enlightened souls?" Amma once asked a group of disciples, and then went on to explain, "They were the souls that had the capacity to connect with the divine. They realized this is not the body anymore; this is divine. For thousands of years when the enlightened souls attained the state of oneness, they found the wisdom of any secret in this universe. One of those secrets is mantras."

Mantra, in the literal Sanskrit translation, means "through the mind"[2]—a definition that illuminates this ancient practice and its significant power in two ways. First, it reminds us that it is not possible to quiet the mind without extreme focus. Through chanting mantras, as the Vedic sages and Siddha masters discovered, a person is able to stop the mind from leaping in many different directions at once and begin to find a profound inner stillness. But the mantra is also considered to be a numinous sound, a hallowed utterance that is simultaneously able to open the mind and body to the boundaryless, shared energy of the universe, while also locating the divine energy within. As it is explained in the Upanishads, there are two forms of divine energy: "the Sound Brahman and the Supreme Brahman. Becoming immersed in the Sound Brahman, one reaches the Supreme Brahman."[3]

The earliest mantras were directly perceived from nature by enlightened masters in a state of awakened listening and then were later composed in ancient Tamil and Sanskrit. These masters became highly attuned to the natural world in order to decipher the various tones that resonate within the vibrations of the universe. Humans evolved, after all, to constantly process the sounds of nature; these sounds exist at the core of auditory perception. Because they derive from nature, mantras provide a primal form of communication with a vast body of knowledge that outstrips language and thought, allowing a person to directly perceive the divine. "Human beings have many different characteristics—some positive and some negative. The divine also has many characteristics, but they are only positive, although in many different aspects: peace, bliss, kindness, love, compassion, mercy, and creativity," as Amma once explained it. "When the human being connects to the energy of the divine in its seed form through mantra, the human being begins to also have those qualities of the divine vibrations spontaneously." This is also when a person has achieved resonance with nature, which occurs, as you may remember, when two objects vibrate at the same frequency.

The ancient mantras were also used as the foundation for the four yogic paths. In fact, the oldest yogic texts and spiritual teachings, collected in the Rigveda, are primarily a teaching of mantra as a path toward obtaining union.[4] The mantras of karma yoga, for instance, were seen as powerful tools for reducing or negating past bad actions. If every action or thought has a vibratory component, it was believed, harmful behavior would result in negative vibrations held in the Akash—or, in our modern understanding, the zero point field—which reverberate back to the one who set them in motion in the first place, like a karmic boomerang. Anandamaya, the bliss sheath, which is related to the element Akash as well as to speech and sound, is believed to hold the seeds of our karma. Vedic philosophy proposes that mantras can pierce and transform this field, modifying those vibrations and, consequently, altering the karmic imprint.

In raja yoga, and more extensively in hatha yoga, where the asanas, or poses, were devised to build discipline through the body, mantras were engaged to do this mentally—creating greater focus, flexibility, and stability in the mind. Once mastered, every asana, and every mantra, becomes a conduit for a greater flow of energy.

Additionally, each of the ancient Sanskrit mantras is constructed to address specific health issues—ranging from anxiety and depression to digestive issues—depending on how the syllables of the mantra stimulate the brain and body, directing prana to particular organs. Medically prescriptive mantras can be given by a qualified practitioner and are often accompanied by specific and complementary herbs to be taken for the ailment. General mantras, such as the chakra mantra, can be used without the oversight of an Ayurvedic practitioner.

The ancient science of mantra has, indeed, proved to be both comprehensive and complex in its design and ability to convey subtle information. There is a musical and mathematical precision inherent in these mantras that has been carefully preserved through history. Even today, children as young as four years old in certain parts of India begin to learn the precise pronunciations and variations of the vast body of Vedic mantras. The exact sounds of the mantras are trusted as ancient wisdom just as the mathematics behind the intricate structures and symmetries in the music of Johann Sebastian Bach is received as an implicit truth in the West. It is possible, though, to formally study the mathematical rigor of mantras. One such study, from *Science of the Sacred: Ancient Perspectives for Modern Science,* compiled by David Osborn,[5] drawing from the Indian monk Bharati Krishna Tirtha Maharaja's book *Vedic Mathematics,* demonstrated that mathematical formulas were often taught within the context of mantras—with each Sanskrit consonant attached to a specific number, allowing for calculations to be done; one of the Vedic sutras even offers a key for deciphering the value of pi to 32 decimal places.

The musical and mathematical intricacies of mantras pertain more to the traditional mantras chanted, often for more than an hour, by those being acculturated in Vedic tradition; however, the bija mantra embodies the same mathematical code and reverberations of nature, just in more concise form. That is the beauty and advantage of the mantra practice—it is not necessary to be a Vedic master to resonate with nature and the universe, and to affect the body and mind. Amma gives a wonderful analogy that Indian masters have cited about the bija mantras: She explains that the seed of a banyan tree is very small, half the size even of a mustard seed, but all of the information needed to grow into an enormous banyan tree—which sometimes reach one hundred feet—is contained in that seed. Similarly, the existence of the whole universe is hiding in the letters of the bija mantra—fittingly also known as a seed mantra.

Remember, though, that even a bija mantra needs to be coupled with an emotional force for it to be fully awakened or "activated." This happens in one of two ways: An enlightened spiritual teacher, someone like Amma, can activate a mantra at the time it is given to a student. Amma, indeed, had activated the chakra mantra when she taught it to me on my pivotal visit to India—after which I felt a sudden expansion in my practice and I began to feel more fluid, less like skin and bones, and more like energy. With this method, a guru, typically associated with a particular yogic tradition, has received a mantra through a lineage of previous teachers and shares it with someone who will bring it forth into the world for healing the body, mind, and spirit. (Amma is a guru within the bhakti yoga tradition.) In this day and age, however, this is a rare occurrence—more often, the path toward activating a mantra is taken by someone who is establishing a practice without a spiritual teacher.

When someone needs to activate her own mantra, it is necessary to establish a regular practice, of course, but, more important, a feeling of love and devotion must infuse the mantra as it is being chanted. This is what my patient Tim did, as I described in the previous chapter, when he began to practice bhakti yoga—chanting the chakra mantra I'd taught him while looking at a picture of Mother Mary, who had served as a symbol of maternal warmth for him as a child. In doing so, he'd not only become unexpectedly aware of his wife's boundless commitment; he'd also started to activate his mantra. It is, as Tim learned, the opening of the heart chakra that ultimately connects us to the divine. This is, in fact, depicted graphically in the Vedic illustration of the heart chakra,[6] which shows the heart symbol sitting in the core of the crown chakra, emphasizing the role of unconditional love as a necessary quality to achieve the higher intelligence, and divine energy, within us.[7]

I should say that bhakti yoga is not the only path for activating a mantra—the other yogic paths are all aimed toward this as well—but bhakti yoga is the most realistic in our hurried modern lives, which is why it is the one that I recommend for my patients. If a person chooses to pursue activation through jnana yoga, for instance, it is a cryptic and arduous journey. I consider Jung's process in writing *The Red Book*[8]—the red leather-bound narrative of his thoughts and imaginative experiences occurring primarily from 1913 to 1917—as an example of a jnana yogic pursuit of, if not specifically an activated mantra, then union in the true Vedic sense of the word. *The Red Book*—or, as Jung called it, *Liber Novus* (Latin for "New Book")—is a chronicle of the Swiss psychologist's willful engagement with his unconscious. Jung deliberately, and daily, evoked a dream state in waking life and then recorded his visions and fantasies.[9] "The years . . . when I pursued the inner images, were the most important time of my life. Everything else is to be derived from this," Jung wrote about this experiment. "It began at that time, and the later details hardly matter anymore. My entire life consisted in elaborating what had burst forth from the unconscious and flooded me like an enigmatic stream and threatened to break me. That was the stuff and material for more than only one life. Everything later was merely the outer classification, scientific elaboration, and the integration into life. But the numinous beginning, which contained everything, was then."[10]

With bhakti yoga, once a person awakens what the Vedic sages call the "Shakti" of the mantra—referring to Shakti, or the divine feminine energy that underlies nature itself—the mantra connects to the universal consciousness, or Brahman. "Since it [the bija] is the seed, when you sow the seed in the soil, it grows," as Amma once eloquently put it. "When you sow the seed mantras in your heart, it grows as a tree with the divine." She also rather specifically and reassuringly explained that an activated mantra, whether chanted by an experienced practitioner or a newcomer, need be practiced for only thirty minutes and "by the thirty-first minute, he will find peace within himself and, when he does it nine days regularly then he will enjoy the bliss." Once we have reached the point of activation in our mantra practice, we can achieve resonance with the vibrations of nature—this energizing of the body, this enlivening of every cell, lasts far beyond the meditative state. "When someone awakes the divine energy," Amma says, "he cannot go back to being negative."

Similarly, it is possible to transfer this divine energy, where it can live on as a continuously positive force. There is, in Hindu culture, a practice of using mantra to charge water—activating it and transforming it into holy water. I mentioned earlier that when I attend the puja ceremonies, Amma distributes the theertham, which is the Sanskrit name for such holy water, giving everyone a spoonful to drink. Theertham, infused as it is with the energy of mantras chanted over it, is believed to be able to help increase the resonance of divine energy in the body, allowing those who receive it to feel healthier and more at peace. Indeed, when I have received theertham from Amma, I have felt an immediate and palpable sense of calm and restoration.

Theertham was also used to bless holy statues as well as homes and offices (and is still used to do this in some parts of India today)—further evidence that mantras were an inseparable part of Vedic life in every aspect. They were used in multiple disciplines—the Ayurvedic medical system, of course, but also vastu shastra, or the architectural system, and Vedic agriculture. Mantras, too, were used to improve all aspects of human activity, not just spiritual pursuits but also commerce, marriage, and education. Many of these customs are still practiced today in India. Before a new business is launched, for example, a special mantra to offer good fortune for it in the future is often chanted in the offices. And, on a particular day once a year, students come to temples to chant a mantra to Saraswati, the goddess of knowledge, to help support their education and quest for wisdom. (My son, too, has done this since we moved to India.)

And as the modern world of yoga begins to shift its attention from physical postures to consciousness, mantra is beginning to emerge with greater popularity in the West. In popular culture, this is reflected in the music of the Deva Premal & Miten Band, who use mantras and instrumental improvisation as the basis for their music—creating global bhakti yoga gatherings in which the audience participates in chanting mantras along with the band, as opposed to traditional concerts. Deva Premal & Miten have sold over a million albums[11] and garnered well-known fans such as the Dalai Lama, Tony Robbins, and Cher. And Cher herself sang the Gayatri mantra, one of the most revered mantras in the Vedas, while riding on a giant mechanical elephant during her 2002 to 2004 Living Proof: The Farewell Tour and then reprised it in her 2017 to 2019 Classic Cher tour.[12]

In a more formal way, Transcendental Meditation (TM), a form of silent bija mantra charged by its lineage of spiritual teachers dating back to ancient Vedic tradition, has steadily grown as a practice in America. It was first popularized in the West by the Indian guru Maharishi Mahesh Yogi during his TM world tours between 1958 and 1965.[13] Interest only increased when, in 1968, the Beatles discovered Maharishi giving a lecture in England and followed him back to Rishikesh, India, to study with him.[14] Since then, the TM movement has strengthened, spearheaded in large part by the film director David Lynch, whose foundation aims to establish a mainstream understanding of the TM program and its positive health effects, as well as pro bono TM instruction to underserved populations.[15] There is also a long list of celebrities—Jerry Seinfeld, Oprah, Lena Dunham, Ellen DeGeneres, and Rupert Murdoch among them—who are self-professed TMers and promote it widely.

Thanks to this celebrity recognition, the health benefits of this particular form of silent bija mantra meditation have been extraordinarily well studied. Just as with ultrasonic and infrasonic waves, the sounds of mantra themselves, even when chanted only within the mind and therefore not ascribed sound or meaning, still act as sound waves and are able to alter vibrations within the body. The mantra recitation of TM has been shown to affect the nervous system, activating frontal and parietal areas of the brain. As such, TM has been shown to reduce clinical depression. Depression causes aspects of the brain to slow down, such as certain parts of the frontal lobe and parietal lobe, which is why "activating" them with meditation is useful in contending with the neurochemistry of this mental health disorder. This has also been clinically demonstrated in a 2010 UCLA study[16] in which participants reported their depressive symptoms nearly halved within three months of starting treatment.

Additionally, a landmark 1978 study published in *Hormones and Behavior* revealed that TM reduces cortisol—the stress hormone—by 30 percent.[17] Similarly, a 1989 meta-analysis conducted by Stanford University of 146 independent studies illustrated that TM is twice as effective at decreasing stress as compared with concentration, contemplation, and other techniques.[18] A 2013 study published in *Military Medicine* showed that active duty U.S. armed forces members previously diagnosed with PTSD who silently chanted a TM mantra for twenty minutes twice a day for two months were also able to reduce their symptoms. In fact, in 2012, the U.S. Department of Defense awarded a $2.4 million grant to the San Diego Veterans Administration Medical Center, in conjunction with the Maharishi University of Management Research Institute, to further study the effect of TM on PTSD in veterans.[19]

More recently, a large body of research has emerged illustrating that TM is effective in combating attention deficit–hyperactivity disorder (ADHD), which is believed to affect a variety of executive functions, including the brain circuitry that governs behavior.[20] Since TM can be easily learned and practiced for only twenty minutes twice a day, and has shown to increase the inhibitory control as well as the stress response in the brain, this practice is becoming a first line intervention for children and adolescents with ADHD. Over the last decade, a meditation program called Quiet Time has been implemented in public schools around the country.[21] According to the David Lynch Foundation, this has resulted in not only a reduction in ADHD symptoms but also an 86 percent decrease in suspensions over two years; a 40 percent lessening of psychological distress, including stress and anxiety; a 10 percent improvement in test scores; and a 65 percent decrease in violent conflict over two years.[22]

There are physiological benefits, too: Research shows that TM lowers blood pressure, reduces the risk of heart attack and stroke, lowers high cholesterol as well as high blood pressure, and reduces mortality rates by almost 50 percent for those who have been practicing for five years.[23] The effect of mantra meditation on heart disease has been proved effective enough, in fact, for the American Academy of Cardiology to recommend it in 2017, as an adjunct treatment, for coronary heart disease.[24]

Beyond the clinical research about TM and bija mantra, there is also a broader body of theoretical research on how sound more generally may affect our biology. To fully understand the radical advances these theories propose, however, we must briefly revisit the idea of electromagnetic fields within the body. As we know, these biofields are physical fields produced by electrically charged particles in motion. They are smooth, continuous fields, extending indefinitely into space, propagated in a wave-like manner, and they transport the type of energy we call electromagnetic radiation, or light. We use the terms *electromagnetic waves*, *radiation*, and *light* interchangeably to refer to the same physical phenomenon: electromagnetic energy.[25]

Historically, we have not understood electromagnetic energy in terms of biology or the effect of its field on biological systems. Questions about consciousness and self-organization had no place in the mechanistic theories of Newton's physics. This had enormous impact on not only how we came to view biology but also how we began to look at ourselves and at the universe.

Perhaps most important, it determined, in explicit and implicit ways, our prevailing medical models. The research that was pursued biases us in terms of what we both focus on and accept in science. (You'll remember the fierce, decades-long dispute Jacques Benveniste sparked with his unconventional study of "water memory.")

But over time, as our biases slowly shift and give way to change, so, too, does the evolution of physics and biology. The electrocardiogram (EKG) and the electroencephalogram (EEG) have become a mainstay of Western diagnostics since their invention in the early 1900s. In neurology, we now also use auditory data of electrical fields generated by muscle contraction when performing an electromyogram (EMG) in the diagnosis of both muscle and peripheral nerve disorders. In these small ways, the medical use and interpretation of electromagnetic fields has become part of our accepted medical system. And yet, despite the fact that we are using endogenous electromagnetic fields as a measurement in Western medicine, we still don't have a model for their role in biology.

After the emergence of quantum physics and the zero point field, researchers have begun to look at field effects in biology, realizing that electromagnetic fields have a further-reaching effect than previously understood. Consequently, biofield science developed to study the fields that the human body emits—both conventionally accepted electromagnetic fields as well as subtler ones—and the ways in which those fields might transmit energy and information to regulate the homeodynamic function of the body, as well as play a role in directing our health processes.

This branch of science has yielded fascinating results, finding, for example, as Drs. Igor Jerman, Robert Leskovar, and
R. Krašovec did in 2012, that every living cell membrane
"has an electric field of very high intensity . . . though of a
rather low voltage . . . one of the basic features of life."[26] This
electric field is what, in 2015, John Hubacher captured when
he expanded on the phantom leaf effect first made famous
by Semyon Kirlian. In 1939, Kirlian photographed what he
believed was the human biofield, or the corona discharge (the
term in physics for an electrical glow on or around a charged
conductor), when he placed photographic paper between elec-
trodes and the skin of his hand and took a photographic image. The resulting pictures indeed showed a luminescent glow
surrounding his hand and fingers. Later, Kirlian adapted the
method to photograph a torn leaf, finding again that he had
captured what he described as an "aura," a luminescent outline of the leaf, even where the missing part had been.

For his updated experiment, Hubacher tore off between 30
and 60 percent of the leaves of plants and, using Kirlian's im-
aging process, took pictures of the remaining leaf sections. A
total of 137 leaves were photographed; of those, 96 showed
the phantom corona discharge outlining even the missing part,
offering a ghostly but coherent image of the whole leaf. This
provided enough statistical evidence to cite the possibility of an
invisible biological field.[27]

Perhaps the most startling finding of all, however, occurred in 2004, when Jiří Pokorný of the Institute of Radio
Engineering and Electronics in the Czech Republic discovered that microtubules (which direct the basic structure of

the cytoskeleton of every cell in the human body) emit their own endogenous electromagnetic fields.[28] This has tremendous significance given that microtubules are critical to basic cellular functions including cell division and regulating intracellular transportation. Moreover, this finding suggests a form of coherent electromagnetic activity throughout the entire body. The endogenous fields of the microtubules would be able to interact with other fields instantaneously within the body as well as retrieve information—an extraordinarily similar view to the Vedic concept of layered sheaths that comprise what we call the biofield—and communicate information on successively deeper levels. (Similarly, we have long known that protein molecules don't have to be in direct contact to exert an effect on each other—the electromagnetic field of one protein influences the spin of another.)

In another astounding turn in biofield science, an enormous amount of research has been conducted to determine how electromagnetic fields might be applied deliberately to the body to affect biological change. One of the more auspicious aspects of these findings is a study on how to stimulate stem cells—an exciting frontier in medicine thanks to their unique ability to regenerate and repair damaged tissue—to become specific cell lines dependent on the type of electromagnetic field exposure given.[29] Most notably, several research groups have reported that electromagnetic field exposure can coax mesenchymal stem cells (those that can differentiate into a variety of cell types, including bone, cartilage, and muscle cells) toward cardiac muscle cell–like and chondrocyte-like (chondrocytes are cells found in cartilage connective tissue) gene expression, suggesting the possibility of reprogramming stem cells toward fates other than their original purpose.[30] This suggests the possibility of a new way to counteract aging and disease through the use of electromagnetic fields—using them to urge stem cells to regenerate damaged tissue.

And in a 1995 study conducted by Betty Sisken, a professor at the Center for Biomedical Engineering at the University of Kentucky, and Janet Walker, a pediatric orthopedic surgeon and professor of pediatric orthopedics at the University of Kentucky School of Medicine, investigating the therapeutic applications of electromagnetic fields for soft-tissue healing, the researchers found specific measurements at which the body responded: 2 Hz associated with nerve regeneration; 10 Hz with ligament healing; 15, 20, and 72 Hz associated with capillary formation and fibroblast proliferation.[31]

In March 2015, in fact, the cover story of *Scientific American* magazine, its headline marching across a person's head and neck with daggers of electricity entering from either side, proposed "Electric Cures: Bioelectronic medicine could create an 'off switch' for arthritis, diabetes and even cancer."[32] Indeed, using devices that emit electrical impulses, now dubbed "electroceuticals," to apply electromagnetic fields as therapeutic interventions may be the "big pharma" of the future.

In essence, science has grown comfortable with the idea that there are electromagnetic fields that shift and communicate inside each of us. I believe, however, that there is biologically relevant information being passed by and to these fields as well. "Bioelectromagnetic research has uncovered a surprising fact.

Extremely low intensity, non-ionizing electromagnetic fields, having even less energy content than the physical thermal noise limit, can produce biological effects," Beverly Rubik wrote in a 2002 piece published in the *Journal of Alternative and Complementary Medicine*.[33] "This means that such extremely low-level fields cannot act energetically on organisms, because the energy content is negligible. Thus, it has been proposed that they are acting informationally." In other words, the thermal energy being produced by these fields is so weak—weaker than even the biological white noise—that we can only conclude that biological information must be transmitted another way.

I believe that a subtler field is carrying this information. Just as the vibration of the molecules that were recorded and exposed to water prompted the water to retain a "memory" of them in Benveniste's 1984 experiment, I believe that biological information is communicated by the vibrational energy of sound.

This is the foundational theory of sonocytology, the field of research created by Dr. James Gimzewski and Andrew Pelling, in which they were able to detect the vibrations of the cell wall and amplify them so that they are audible to the human ear, revealing that every cell in our bodies has a unique song. Gimzewski theorizes playing back the amplified frequencies of specific cells could be used as a diagnostic tool for identifying healthy cells versus injurious ones—as well as the potential ability to play the destructive sounds of rogue cells back to them greatly amplified, so that they implode and are destroyed. Gimzewski and Pelling have since also proposed the idea of "biomusic" where bio-information "sounds" from cells, tissues, and organs are targeted toward cell populations to enhance the regulation of a variety of biological processes including differentiation, stem cell reprogramming, and the maintenance of biological homeostasis. Such biomusic may be able to transmit the information of the biofield and could be implemented as a strategy to support cell therapy and regenerative medicine. They are currently looking to patent this technology.[34]

It seems the use of sound—both audible and inaudible—and its resulting influence on biology through its impact on electromagnetic fields may be a fundamental form of communication within the body that has been, until recently, overlooked. This communication system and its resulting influence on the endogenous electromagnetic fields of the human body may not only be more essential, it may also be faster and more dynamic than even the nervous system. The research—and possibilities it raises—are so significant that I am in complete agreement with Beverly Rubik, a pioneer of biofield science, who recommended that we need a "human energy project," something similar to the Human Genome Project, with funding and the full commitment of the scientific community. [35]

If, indeed, sound shares quantum information capable of altering electromagnetic fields and producing shifts in the body, this would offer a modern biological model for the science of mantras. If this is true, it would not only revolutionize medicine but completely change the way in which we view life itself.

For the great, enlightened masters, in particular the Siddhas, consciousness and energy meet in the realm of vibration. The vibration that shapes and transforms the physical world is called sound, whether it is audible or not. The Siddhas understood life as a system of resonance—finding a synchronistic chord not only in nature but also with the divine. Sound was the key to connecting with this energy. As such, they created self-generated vibrations in the form of mantras. These were drawn from the infinite field of vibrations held within space—what they called the Akash and what a quantum physicist would call the ZPF. Our modern scientific discoveries in quantum physics and the biofield seem to be consistently leading us back to what these ancient masters already knew: *The universe is singing.*

9

THE SIDDHAS

Science without religion is blind; and religion without science is lame.

—ALBERT EINSTEIN

Looking back, it seems to me that I had been traveling a winding path interwoven by circumstance and happenstance until finally, somewhere along the way, the two converged into the straight, determined passage of fate. It was an unexpected twist in my mother's life, and then in my own, that landed me in Norma's bright, plant-filled home in Southern California, sitting at rapt attention as she whispered that alluring bija mantra into my ear. I was too young then—my life not yet unfolded enough—to put this experience into context. I took the mantra for what it seemed to be: a wonderful and mysterious sound; an instruction from my mother, and Norma, to silently chant it every day; a place to retreat in my mind that offered a complete escape from the world and anything within it that felt overpowering.

By the time that I had reached medical school, however, I had a clear sense of myself, and my connection to the divine energy underlying everything. So it was that when I came to do my neurology rotation for the first time, I was hit with a bolt of certainty that *this* was my field, a place for me within the world of medicine. I was, and still am, fascinated by the brain as a discrete organ—by the complexity of its circuitry and the elegance of its organization—but I also sensed that there might be something more for me in this discipline if I pursued it on my own terms. I had an instinct that the nervous system, responsible for so much of the communication within the body, might be the window to something more expansive, something revolutionary. I thought if I could understand not only the brain but also the mind and consciousness, and merge this knowledge with the mystic insights of my mantra meditation practice, I might be able to explain the place with no boundaries, with its infinite sense of possibility and renewal, that I'd been visiting since I was a child. This convergence of science and metaphysics was the black box of medicine for me, and I desperately wanted to decipher it.

Medical school was the first in a series of events and opportunities in my career that I've recounted throughout this book: taking over the neurology practice at Scripps and reconstructing it as an integrative practice, implementing mantra in the lives of my patients, meeting Amma in India, and, later, her request that I become the unit head of the Ayurvedic and Siddha medicine center in Tamil Nadu. Now, in hindsight, I can see clearly the moment my curving path became a decisive one. I was visiting Amma—it was my third trip to Peedam, the spiritual retreat located in Tamil Nadu, in 2012. We were at her house, having a casual conversation—as casual, that is, as it ever feels between a spiritual teacher and student.

"What is it that you want, Kulreet?" Amma asked me out of the blue.

I felt an electric sense of opening. I sensed that I could say anything then—to be the most famous physician in the world; constant happiness; eternal life—and it would happen, in the same mysterious way that Amma's advice, even when it seems far-fetched, turns out to be correct. I felt time slow. My surroundings became abundantly clear, as if the world were pixelated. Logic dropped away; I became pure instinct.

"Surrender," I heard myself say.

The term *Siddha*, in Sanskrit, refers to one who has attained perfection in both the physical and spiritual realms—meaning one who has achieved ultimate enlightenment. Siddhas, sometimes called *Siddhars* (from the ancient language of Tamil Nadu), were wandering spiritual adepts of the early ages believed to be descended from the Dravidians, the majority population across the Indian subcontinent before the second millennium.[1] Incidentally, Sanskrit and Tamil are among the world's oldest classical languages. The exact date of the first appearance of the Siddhas is unknown. Some say they have existed since the beginning of history, while others argue their transcendent powers place them outside of the framework of time and space.

Indeed, the Siddhas are believed to have eight supernatural powers:[2]

1. *Aṇimā*: reducing one's body to the size of an atom
2. *Mahimā*: expanding one's body to an infinitely large size
3. *Garimā*: becoming infinitely heavy
4. *Laghimā*: becoming almost weightless
5. *Prāpti*: ability to be anywhere at will throughout all of the dimensions of creation
6. *Prākāmya*: realizing whatever one desires
7. *Īśiṭva*: supremacy over nature
8. *Vaśiṭva*: control of the forces of nature; dominion over the five elements

Still other historians assert that, even taking the mythic and miraculous qualities of the Siddhas out of the equation, it is difficult to place them on a definitive timeline because their movements from one country to the next are recorded only in their own literature and not in other sources, making it impossible to verify.[3] The *concept*, however, of these spiritualists can be traced back to its earliest mentions in writings during the Sangam period (500 BC to AD 500).[4]

Because the Siddhas seeded their knowledge throughout the world, they are not associated with one particular society or religion. Some of the Tamil Nadu Siddhas hail from around the small rural village where I now live, but there are also similar traditions outside of India influenced by the Siddhas, such as the Eight Immortals of ancient China, a legendary group who also possessed divine powers.[5] Still, the Tamil Nadu Siddhas are considered one of the primal, uninterrupted lineages of the Siddhas, with continuous, albeit closely guarded, records of their writings, including the palm leaves that Amma now has in her possession, still in existence.

The Tamil Nadu Siddhas were (and are—there are still reportedly Siddhas in existence) preternaturally intelligent and perceptive; their insights dominate ancient Tamil teachings. They devised elaborate systems of philosophy, math, science, and medicine, all informed by a profound understanding of nature. The palm leaf manuscripts detail the many theories of Siddha medicine, as well as the herbal formulations and instructions for metallurgy (an alchemical process used to transform metals and metallic elements, such as mercury, for medicinal purposes).[6] The palm leaves also include an account of the root of its long oral history: Lord Shiva—the Hindu deity believed to represent pure consciousness—explained the Siddha systems to his wife Parvati; she, in turn, offered this wisdom to her son, Lord Murugan, who taught all that he knew to his disciple Agastya, considered, in Tamil Hindu traditions, to be the first sage to perfect his knowledge of the natural and spiritual worlds. For this reason, Agastya is regarded as the father of Siddha medicine; he passed his wisdom on to eighteen Siddhas and, from there, quietly spread their knowledge to human beings across the world.

Throughout history, two of the strongest characteristics of the Siddhas have been compassion and secrecy. They have tremendous empathy for the plight of humanity and a strong desire to relieve it; they have also always lived on the outer boundaries of history even as they have shaped it. The

Siddhas have an abiding reverence and respect for the universe, taking genuine pleasure in deciphering how humanity could benefit from the mighty offerings of the natural world. And yet to reach this realm of intelligence and generosity requires incredible self-control, spiritual stamina, rigor, and introspection. The Siddhas believe that if one can gain mastery over the mind and body, it is possible also to collaborate with the phenomena of nature. The mind, and the power of concentration achieved in mantra meditation, is one of the most direct ways to access Brahman. The Siddhas teach that the only things we will carry beyond this life are our character and our experience—and the knowledge gained from both—so it should be our highest priority to cultivate our own divine natures.

In Sanskrit, the word *tapas* means "inner heat"—this word is used to describe the physical and mental austerities practiced to achieve spiritual powers.[7] The Siddhas undergo severe tapas, sacrificing everything they have materially and intellectually, to strip themselves of their earthbound desires and attachments. Some Siddhas, as it has been passed on through oral history, lived in caves not tall enough to stand up in, keeping a vow of silence for more than a year.[8] Other stories recount intense fasting and yogic practices. To reach ultimate yoga—true surrender to and communion with Brahman—requires a complete and fiery dissolution of the ego. The often harsh and unconventional teachings of the Siddhas were meant to test, to push beyond seeming possibility. "The Siddhas are the cyclonic storms," as Palpandian describes them in his book *Siddhas: Masters of the Basics*, "shaking and uprooting trees!"[9]

I didn't fully know what I meant by "surrender" when I said it to Amma that day. I knew only that, once I'd uttered the word, it was my truest, deepest desire. But it was an answer delivered by instinct, and therefore its full significance lay somewhere out of reach. I had no idea what surrender would come to represent in my life. In that moment my rational self and my romantic self thought I meant I'd give over my whole heart and mind in pursuit of my field—with my superhero cape pulled around me and the comfort and structure of the life I'd built in California bolstering me.

That part of the dream—the first layer, or sheath, of surrender—did occur initially. After I returned from my visit to Amma in 2012, my career began to shift, and I began to garner the accolades that I'd thought I'd wanted to define my professional rise: television appearances, a book deal, cofounder of a medical company, an increasing salary. All of this success was set against the backdrop of an idyllic home life: I lived with my husband and son in a beautiful house on the beach in San Diego. My extended family, including my mother, lived near us; we all routinely gathered at the beach and family dinners. It did feel magically like I was easily enjoying the best of both worlds—a thriving career and fulfilling home life—until, that is, I came to understand what I had really meant by surrender.

When I chose to move to India, I knew that I would be giving up living in proximity to my beautiful extended family and the prestige of the career I'd built, along with the salary that had come with it. I knew that I'd be living in a rural village with few of the modern amenities that I took for granted in America. I suppose, too, that I knew I would be entering a predominantly male-dominated culture in which I'd struggle to be viewed as equal. But what I hadn't realized was how I'd be tested beyond all of this—feeling at times as if the price of entry into this mysterious world would be my sanity—by Amma herself.

When I was first meant to move to India, for example, I understood that my work with Amma would begin in May of 2018, affording me the time I needed to finish up seeing patients at the Chopra Center as well as to tie up other logistical loose ends. But, when my husband visited Peedam in January of that year, Amma told him out of the blue that she wanted me to come in March. It wasn't clear whether this would be for a visit or the beginning of my tenure in India. Amma remained steadfastly vague on this front. I scrambled to move to India earlier, with no idea as to whether I'd be returning to California again or not. One day, walking into the Vishnu temple, I ran into the director of the hospital who mentioned to me that Amma had told him I had moved to India now. Well, that settled that. Next, Amma told me I would start by working in the hospital as a neurologist—which left me dumbfounded because I most certainly hadn't uprooted my whole life and moved to India only to go back to practicing Western medicine. I did so for a time, and was eventually able to launch my outpatient Ayurvedic center within the hospital. Each step of the way the plan has not been what I thought it would be and the bar for surrender has been raised just a little bit higher every time.

I admit I am not facing the same physical austerities of the original lineage of students studying under a Siddha master, but from a modern-day standpoint, I have gone through my own series of deaths of identity. "Don't give up," I remind myself daily of the Siddhas' advice in undergoing their own harsh and unconventional teachings, "but transcend."[10]

Many of the Siddhas' revelations and findings on the subject of health and medicine are written in poetic Tamil verse on the palm leaves that Amma guards. In them, there are four main methods of treatment described: mantra, mani (metallurgy, or the use of gems and metals for healing), varma (application of specific pressure points for healing), and aushadha (herbs and minerals for healing).

I have focused on the first over the last year—mantra and sound medicine—and am now beginning to learn about varma and aushadha. Since much of the instruction comes from oral tradition, I'm never certain when Amma is formally teaching me because the lessons are dispersed through seemingly conversational points that, only later in my meditation, begin to unravel as deep truths about the nature of life. Recently, for example, I was walking with Amma in her garden after lunch and she noted that one of the herbs used in Siddha medicine was drying nearby in the sun on a piece of cloth. She told me that the preparation of this particular herb is critical because there is one part of the herb that is poisonous but the other part offers a very potent cure for the mind. She asked me to take a look at the herb in her garden; I did. Then we moved on with our conversation and our walk. But, in the weeks following that passing conversation, in my meditations as well as my visits with patients, I began to understand more about this part of Siddha medicine—more about the herb itself but also more about the notion of poison and panacea—or dark and light, and the underlying unity to these two extremes. I realized that this concept plays a big role in Siddha medicine more broadly; that is, many of the herbal formulations are so potent because the Siddhas learned to use herbs that were extremely dangerous, given their poisonous potential, and draw from them their opposites, or their curative properties.

This, too, is consistent with the Siddha practice. As Palpandian notes in *Siddhas: Masters of the Basics,* "the genuine initiation is the Master sharing with the disciple the very sap of his living experience . . . This way the Master shares no conceptual theories but shares Himself."[11] It is similar, too, to the approach I took in developing my Ayurvedic practice, in that much of my life experience with mantra meditation helped to inform my expertise, but approaching Siddha medicine in this way has been much more intense and has required a greater degree of internal alchemy.

Internal and external alchemy are elemental parts of Siddha training. The Siddha use of the word *alchemy* is different, though, from our understanding in the West— which, ironically, emerged in large part from Isaac Newton's obsession with this ancient branch of philosophy and his pursuit of the Philosopher's Stone, a formula he believed would transform base metal into gold.[12] The Siddhas consider internal alchemy to be the rugged preparation of the individual mind and spirit, the ascetic and yogic transformation they achieve through such acts as fasting, profound purification therapies, living in solitary confinement, and, most particularly, mantra meditation. Their goal was to transmute the consciousness of a person from the limited and conditioned mind to the unlimited perspective of the Self—to forge union with Brahman.

Internal alchemy is necessary before the knowledge of external alchemy—a process that includes taking complex herbal formulas and purification therapies—can be shared. Without first preparing the mind and spirit, the human body cannot properly accept the herbs—either there will be no transformation or the challenge it presents to the mind will lead to psychological disorders. The concept of external alchemy, as the Siddhas portray it, is more complex than it seems. The ultimate goal of external alchemy is immortality. But it does not simply mean becoming ever younger and more vital, extending one's life forever. It means achieving immortality through yoga, through union with the divine through the human biofield. It results in becoming one with infinite consciousness. In this sense, the Siddhas are free from the cycle of birth and death; in transcending the body they are soul in its purest energetic form and can voluntarily incarnate in human bodies in order to help the world progress.

One of the purposes of the external alchemical process is known as Kaya Kalpa,[13] which can bring physical rejuvenation—rendering a person ageless—and also purify the body and mind. Given the highly evolved nature of the Tamil Nadu Siddhas, the motivation behind Kaya Kalpa was not to discover a youth elixir but to stretch their years on earth in order to achieve enlightenment in this lifetime, avoiding the need for reincarnation.

The Indian saint and teacher Maharishi Mahesh Yogi once explained in a lecture that the human body, in its coarse and dense state, is primarily kaphic in nature—composed of the elements of water and earth—and that as we reincarnate our more evolved bodies eventually are made from a substance that is primarily akashic (or etheric) in nature. But to attain this ethereal body requires purification on every level—physical, emotional, psychological, and spiritual; this is a part of the ultimate process of Kaya Kalpa.[14]

Kaya Kalpa is taught even today in the Siddha medical colleges, many of them run under the Indian government universities; while students aren't taught how to enact the process, they nevertheless learn of its potential and existence in history. These academic institutions of Siddha medicine developed only in the last fifty years, initiated by the Indian government in an effort to bring Siddha medicine into the mainstream. Additionally, in 2001, to prohibit bioprospecting and unethical patents, India set up the Traditional Knowledge Digital Library,[15] a repository of 223,000 formulations of various systems of medicine in India—Ayurveda and Siddha medicine among them—and, in 2005, the National Institute of Siddha,[16] committed solely to the research and study of Siddha medicine, was established. The Ministry of AYUSH (Ayurveda, Yoga and Naturopathy, Unani, Siddha and Homeopathy),[17] a governmental body tasked with education and research within these fields of alternative medicine, was created in 2014. And, in addition to the public Siddha medicine universities, there are now five private Siddha medical schools in Tamil Nadu as well as one in the state of Kerala (the main state of Ayurveda in India).[18]

The academic setting for Siddha medicine offers a different kind of tutelage, certainly, than the ancient tradition of guru-disciple learning. In these schools, professors offer the history of Siddha medicine, following textbooks that mimic Western medical education's focus on anatomy, physiology, and pathology. The ancient Siddhas also taught these subjects, but within a broader, holistic perspective that included the knowledge of the divine Self and the process for attainment of yoga (union).

"That which cures physical ailments is medicine; that which cures psychological ailments is medicine," the Siddha master Tirumular wrote of the Siddha ability not only to cure the body but to merge with Brahman. "That which prevents ailments is medicine; that which bestows immortality is medicine." For the Siddhas, the spiritual path was also a scientific approach to regain consciousness of their true natures. Here, beyond even Anandamaya, or the ZPF, they encountered oneness with Brahman and discovered an infinite amount of energy with the capacity to not only heal but also to bring them into a state of unity with the laws governing nature.

The Yajurveda, the Veda primarily composed of mantras for worship rituals, states: "As is the atom, so is the universe."[19] This was a core principle of the Siddhas: Man is nothing but the universe in miniature, containing the five elements. In the few works that have been translated from Tamil by the Siddhas—in addition to the writings I am beginning to translate with a colleague here, a graduate of Siddha medical school who is fluent in ancient Tamil—there are, indeed, references to the quantum nature of reality with descriptions of the oneness of the universe and the inseparability of our experiences that are similar to those of quantum physics.

Just as the theoretical physicist Max Planck held that wholeness must be introduced in physics as in biology and German physicist Niels Bohr asserted the significance of complementarity—the concept that two contrasting theories, such as the wave and particle theories of light, may be able to fully explain a set of phenomena but separately explain only an aspect of it—was paramount in biology,[20] the Siddhas also proposed that subatomic relationships could advance a wider understanding of the biology of the body and the universe. In AD 1000, Siddha Tirumular wrote in his poetic treatise on spirituality, ethics, astronomy, and Siddha medicine, *Tirumantiram*, of pathi, what would be understood as the neutron today, representing the divine aspect of creation; the pass, or proton, illustrating the human ego; and pasam, or the electron, as being indicative of the material world. The properties that Tirumular described for each of these subatomic particles correlates to our modern physics understanding; in this sense, they are two different languages of science describing the same thing.

The Siddha system of healing not only created an understanding of biology as a union between mind, body, and Brahman, but it also contained detailed information about bones, tissue, blood, organs, and hormones. All of this was intuited, and mapped out, by the Siddhas without ever dissecting a human being. They were able to use their keen, transcendent perceptions by piercing all five of the sheaths of the biofield—going beyond even the final layer, Anandamaya, the seat of sound, where consciousness and vibration first meet. This is why mantra meditation is at the core of Siddha medicine. Mantra represents a purposeful gesture toward the inherent, vibratory natural world, a way of communicating through resonance with the universe and the divine.

One of the reasons it is so difficult to find any written records of the lives of the Siddhas, outside of what they themselves wrote, is because, in addition to their tradition of deep secrecy, how does one write about the lives of Immortal Masters? When were they born? When did they die? When they shift from one body to the next—as in the case of Siddha Bogar, who is said to have taken on the appearance of a Chinese man to bring the teaching of Taoism as Lao Tzu for two hundred years before returning to India—how do you accommodate for the continued identity of that Siddha in a new body?

My life in Tamil Nadu has required so much more than the surrender of comforts and security, more even than letting go of my ego and attachments; it has also meant abandoning a recognizable framework of reality. This is what makes it so difficult to write about the Siddhas; it begs the reader, too, to surrender in this way. And I know—believe me I *know*—how difficult it is to relinquish the familiar world in this way.

But I have also found immense, almost unspeakable, reward coupled with such difficulty. I'm not a Siddha, nor even a Siddha physician—though I do hope to one day achieve this.

At this point, I'm essentially a Siddha medicine observer and journalist, the only Western physician I'm aware of who has been brought into direct experience with their secret methods and well-guarded knowledge and with permission to write about it. There is very little I haven't given up of my old life to learn about sound medicine here—but I also consider this to be part of the beauty and strength of my experience.

Not long after Amma had asked me what I truly wanted—and I instinctively responded with "surrender"—I had a dream. Amma and I were walking through a white house with many different rooms. We kept moving forward, through each one. "Not this room, not this room," Amma kept saying as we walked, until finally she brought me to the last room of the house and guided me toward an Indian man with bright, intense eyes and a long, dark beard. Without saying a word, he took his right hand and smashed it into the middle of my forehead, my third eye.

After moving to Tamil Nadu, I learned about Agastya, father of Siddha medicine. Later I came across a picture of him in a book—warm, brown eyes, hair brought into a knot at the top of his head, a long triangular beard. In an instant, I realized *he* was the man from my dream. Such is the mystery and logic of Siddha medicine; as long as I am open to it, I believe that I will learn more about the natural world and the conventions of medicine than I ever knew possible.

The Siddhas determined the laws underlying space, time, and atoms through the use of divine vibrations—or sound. This is why mantra meditation is at the core of Siddha medicine. Mantra represents a purposeful gesture toward the inherent, vibratory natural world, a way of communicating through resonance with the universe and the divine.

As it is outlined in nāda yoga, there are four stages of speech. The first, Vaikhari, are the fundamental sounds that can be heard by the human ear, such as speech and song. The second is Madhyama, meaning "in the middle"; this is a bit subtler than Vaikhari, a whisper that just barely registers as audible. Pashyanti is next: This exists in the deeper levels of the mind and is made up of mental sounds, like words in a dream or a silently chanted mantra. The last is Para Nāda, which literally translates as "transcendental" or "beyond." This level of sound has the highest vibration frequency and, as such, is not a sound that can be perceived within human consciousness. This is a realm of super-consciousness, indescribable by language. This corresponds with the merged condition of the mind with Brahman. It is the Self's own natural language, reverberating in silence, and it is in this state that the Siddhas perceived the first mantras and the reality of all of creation.

I have lived in India for two years now. The further I have delved into the ancient Vedic and Siddha traditions, plumbing the depths of their knowledge about medicine generally and sound in particular, the more I have enriched my own mantra practice. Under the instruction of Amma, I have, in many ways, given up a familiar sense of self-orientation in order to open to the lessons of the Siddhas and sound. It has been mystifying, frustrating, and, at times, frightening, but I have also come to inhabit sound beyond body, mind, and creation in a way I couldn't have otherwise understood was possible. *And I have learned that, borne out of silence, we are the love song of the universe.*

10

YOUR MANTRA
MEDITATION PRACTICE

Beginning any new health practice can be daunting, and starting a daily mantra meditation is no different. My patients are often reluctant for a variety of reasons—they don't understand how to do it, they don't have the time, they do not believe it will work—but once they finally clear the series of hurdles they seemed compelled, initially, to put before themselves, they're inevitably grateful to have incorporated a meditation practice into their lives. There are other meditation techniques that also promote health and well-being—such as focused concentration and self-inquiry—but they're more challenging and not accessible to everyone. What is particularly beneficial about the mantras I'll introduce you to here is that they provide both a mental and a physical way to stay grounded in the moment, and they're among the easiest meditations to master if you find you have trouble reining in a wandering mind.

Mantra meditation is one of the most accessible, affordable, versatile, and potent forms of sound medicine. You can
use different mantras at various points of your life to treat
conditions or circumstances as they arise. As I've explored
throughout this book, sound is a very complex tool—the
mysteries of which we are still unraveling. As with other
forms of medicine, it makes a biological impression on your
body. As we move into the twenty-first century, I believe we
will see that sound medicine has the capacity to launch a new
field of healing that is not only risk free, but also affordable
to everyone. For this reason, we must continue to build the
bridge between the ancient Indian understanding of the science of mantras and our modern recognition of the power of
sound and its ability to heal.

I want to be clear: These suggestions are intended to enhance
your practice, but they are *not* the be-all and end-all. My advice
here is meant to make a practice more comfortable or to inspire you if you are having trouble getting started or feel stalled
out. But once you've found the right mantra—one that not
only resonates with your body and mind but also reflects the
thought or message you'd like to hold within yourself as well
as project into the world—it will extend a feeling of physical
calm and spiritual fulfillment. You don't need the perfect space
or an elaborate altar or a set of crystals to reach the reservoir
of stillness and peace that exists within you. A mantra practice
can be done anywhere, anytime, under any circumstances. The
dignity and power of this practice is that, ultimately, it requires
only a mantra and your mind.

SETTING UP YOUR MANTRA PRACTICE

FIND YOUR SPACE

Eventually, you'll develop the skills to practice mantra meditation anywhere, but in the beginning it's a good idea to dedicate a space to your practice at home or at work. When you meditate, you generate the energy of the mantra that you're chanting and release it into your environment. This permeates the area and supports you in continuing your practice. For this reason, even if the space doesn't feel right at the start—maybe it's not roomy enough, or it's not peaceful enough—the routine and energy dispersed by your mantra practice will alter your sense of this place, ultimately drawing you to it with the promise of the serenity and composure you feel every time you enter it.

You can dedicate an entire room to your meditation practice, but even a corner of your bedroom or another room will do. The only requirements are that the space be quiet and uncluttered; it should be somewhere you feel safe, and where you know you will not be disturbed during your practice. It's also important that you are able to dim the lights in this space. If you don't have a dimmer or a small side lamp, then turn the overhead off and light a candle. If it's too bright, the light will stimulate you, even with your eyes closed. A little sign for the door is also useful: MEDITATION IN PROGRESS or a simple DO NOT DISTURB. It is also helpful to add anything that will make your practice more comfortable, such as a cushion or a yoga mat.

As I was growing up, there was a prayer room in our house where I could practice my meditation. But, over the years, I have also created lovely and functional meditation spaces in the bunk bed of my dorm room, under a tree during my neurology residency, and in a corner of my office when I first started practicing as a neurologist.

CREATE AN ALTAR

Although your "mantra zone" should be relatively open and uncluttered, you might like to add an altar or even just one or two objects that you find meaningful. This will help bring a sense of personal inspiration to your space and your practice. You can add anything from incense to a favorite piece of jewelry or flowers to a picture that promotes a feeling of love and devotion. This is your practice, so you get to choose just what works for you. There are no tried-and-true rules except that any object in your space feels inspiring to you and you will be in comfort while you meditate.

Sometimes my patients ask me to suggest things they might add to their altar or use for their mantra practice that are customary to a mantra practice. These are, of course, not necessary, but the following items can be beneficial in helping a practitioner who wants more of a sense of a traditional practice.

Mala beads. First created in India three thousand years ago, these are traditionally used to help keep count during mantra meditations—*mala* is Sanskrit for "meditation garland." Usually these necklaces have 108 beads strung together and one "guru" bead, which is larger than all the others; there are, however, some that are made of 54 or 27 beads for shorter meditations. To use these, hang the guru bead on the middle finger of the right hand and, while breathing and chanting, use your thumb to count each bead, starting with the guru bead, pulling them toward you along the way. Do this until you've fully traveled around the mala. Once you've reached the guru bead, you can repeat the process. I find that mala beads can also offer a tactile support during meditation as well. Rudraksha malas are the most commonly used; I myself use these beads in my meditations. These are made from the seed of a Rudraksha tree and are considered sacred to Shiva, who, as you now know, is the masculine principle of silent consciousness underlying all of nature. There are other types of mala beads that can be used as well: crystal and tulsi/holy basil (made from the woody stem of the tulsi bush), among them. Other religious traditions have similar practices, such as the Catholic rosary beads used to count the component prayers.

Crystals. These have taken on a New Age sheen, but there is actually a scientific basis to using them. Quartz crystals are considered one of the most beneficial for meditation because of their strong energetic properties; they help to bring clarity and focus to the mind. Another good crystal for beginners is the rose quartz, which is believed to subtly lift the heart to higher frequencies, cultivating devotion and unconditional love. When choosing a crystal, it's important to trust your intuition. Choose the one that draws you to it with its energy.

Deity meditation. Each deity has at least one mantra associated with him or her. Sometimes a specific mantra is used with the hope of achieving the qualities associated with a particular deity. For example, you may chant to the elephant-headed Hindu god Ganesha, known as the Remover of Obstacles, with the mantra "Om Gam Ganapataye Namaha." You may hang a picture of this deity or simply hold the image in your mind. You could also use a picture or image of a spiritual figure such as the Buddha or even someone from your life—whatever or whomever will inspire a feeling of unconditional love.

ATTEND TO YOUR POSTURE

Now that you've set up your space, you need to find the best position to practice in. Again, there are no rules here, but there are a few techniques that may assist in deepening your practice while also maintaining the most effective posture for your well-being. Sitting or standing with proper postural alignment, even while not meditating, is vital for our health generally, as it reduces stress and strain on the body. The most important thing to remember, whether you're sitting on a chair or cross-legged on the floor, is to maintain a straight spine. If you're sitting on a cushion or directly on the floor, Padmasana, or lotus position, in which the legs are crossed and feet rest on the thighs, is the traditional posture for meditation. This is great if you can manage it, but not everyone can—it requires a great deal of flexibility and strength, and people typically experience discomfort unless they have already cultivated a regular hatha yoga practice. It's also fine to sit cross-legged in the regular way. If you choose this position, it's a good idea to change the leg on top from one meditation to the next. This also prevents you from compressing a nerve located around the outer part of the calf just below the knee. Sitting on a chair for meditation is just as effective and often is the best position for beginners getting used to a practice. Be certain to sit upright in the chair, though, and maintain the curve of your spine, with your chin tucked just a bit and with both of your feet flat on the floor. Imagine an invisible string running from the top of your head to the ceiling that's helping keep your body aligned. It can be helpful to sit on the edge of the chair or place a pillow behind you for back support. Keep your hands on your thighs or in your lap and let your palms be relaxed, facing up or down.

START WITH SIMPLE STRETCHING

If you're strapped for time, you can skip this step, but if you have five minutes to spare, I highly recommend some gentle stretching to start. Unless you're already as flexible as a pretzel, it can be hard to stay in a seated pose for an extended period of time. Nothing interrupts the flow of a mantra meditation more than being distracted by a sore back or popping knees or the sensation of tight, tense hips.

Three good moves to try are:

THE YOGA SQUAT (MALASANA)
To open up your inner hip.

- Stand with your feet slightly wider than hip-distance apart. Pivot your feet so that your toes are wider than your heels.
- Bend your knees deeply and squat down until your hips are lower than your knees, a few inches off the floor.

- Bring your palms together in front of your chest and press your elbows into the inside of your knees.
- Hold this pose for 30 to 60 seconds, or the equivalent of about 5 to 10 breaths. To get out of the pose, either lean back to sit on your butt or push back up to standing.

STANDING FORWARD FOLD (UTTANASANA)

To stretch out your lower back and spine, which will make sitting more comfortable.

- Stand with your feet hip-width apart.
- Gently bend down from your hips and place your hands on your knees and stop for a deep breath. Inhale and extend your spine, then exhale and continue to reach for the floor. Reach for your toes, but if you cannot reach your toes, reach as far down your leg as possible and grasp your legs at that place.
- Hold this pose and continue to breathe deeply for 5 to 10 breaths. If you're feeling a lot of tension in your lower back or the backs of your legs, you can gently sway from side to side.
- Roll up slowly.

LUNGE POSE (ANJANEYASANA)

To open up the back, hip, and groin muscles.

- Get on your hands and knees, your spine parallel to the floor and your arms and thighs perpendicular.

- Move your left knee forward, putting your left lower leg on the ground with your heel close to your groin.
- Extend your right leg behind you with your right knee facing down to the ground.
- Draw your pubic bone down toward the ground while simultaneously lifting your chest up, sweeping your arms out to the sides and up, perpendicular to the floor.
- Slowly tilt your head back and look up.
- Hold for 5 to 10 breaths, release the pose, and repeat on the other side.

For those who have more time to dedicate to a regular yoga asana practice, I recommend ten minutes of the sun salutation series of stretches (also known as Surya Namaskar)—which can easily be found on YouTube and are taught at every yoga studio. These are best to do in the morning, if possible.

CALM YOUR MIND THROUGH BREATHING

Mantra meditation also involves pranayama, the formal practice of controlling our breath, which is linked to prana or life force. Research shows that slowed breathing can reduce symptoms of depression and anxiety. This may be because breathing meditations have been shown to increase prefrontal asymmetry, which is linked to elevating the mood. Practicing breathing techniques, too, can lower blood pressure and heart rate, especially in people who already have hypertension. I suggest that my patients engage in slow breathing for a few minutes before they begin their mantra meditation, as a way to settle the mind. In particular, I recommend alternate nostril breathing, or Nadi Shodhana. This is a very simple yet dynamic technique. It carries health benefits as well: It improves memory and cognition by balancing the left and right hemispheres of the brain and can also help with stress-related symptoms such as chronic headaches.

Here's how to do it:

- Use the thumb of your right hand to close your right nostril.
- Fully inhale through your left nostril.
- Close your left nostril with the index or ring finger of your right hand, and exhale through your right nostril.
- Inhale through your right nostril, then close it and exhale through your left nostril.
- Continue repeating, alternating nostrils for each inhale and exhale.

Once you've become comfortable with alternate nostril breathing, you can change your breath ratio: Rather than breathe in an equal breath ratio—equal inhale, equal exhale—change the amount of time for one of them. When you emphasize inhaling, you activate your sympathetic nervous system, which raises heart rate and blood pressure, boosting alertness and stimulating the body. Focus more on this side if these are the qualities you'd like to achieve. When you focus on exhaling, you activate the parasympathetic nervous system, which slows down your heartbeat and relaxes your circulation, nervous system, and digestive system. Irrespective of the side you concentrate on—boosting your alertness or calming yourself down—this exercise leads to an overall feeling of relaxation and well-being.

ESTABLISH A REGULAR SCHEDULE

The nuts and bolts of how and when you practice mantra is less important than simply making it a priority to perform it daily. As with any habit, you've got to practice regularly in order for it to become second nature. Ideally, you will do it at the same time each day as well, because your body will get used to this schedule and begin to gravitate naturally toward the meditative state at that time on its own.

The biggest challenge most people face when it comes to establishing a mantra practice is simply finding the time. It's tough to drop work, family, and even social responsibilities—you're already juggling so much at once, you can't even imagine the look on your partner's face when you tell them you need to push your dinner date back half an hour so you can go home to meditate. I recommend appointing mantra time, just as you would schedule in your workouts. Remember, the quality of the practice is better than quantity. The minimal recommended time to have a significant effect is twenty to thirty minutes a day. If you have time, twenty minutes twice a day helps to maintain the effects of the mantra throughout a twenty-four-hour period. That being said, it's more important to start a mantra meditation than to aim for an unrealistic time requirement in the beginning. If that means you have only five minutes for a mantra practice, then start with five minutes. For most people, the benefits that come from regular mantra practice become the greatest motivation to sustain it. Over time, most people feel that they are becoming more efficient at work and experiencing fewer conflicts—from that perspective, their mantra practice actually saves them more time than it takes each day.

And on those days when you don't even have five minutes? No problem. Family emergencies and work deadlines are part of life. But no matter what the reason for the time crunch, I guarantee you that you still have one minute. Set your phone timer, lock your office door, and get into your mantra pose. Try to squeeze in these one-minute moments throughout your day: when you wake up, before sitting down to start work, during lunch, right before you get in your car and head home in rush hour traffic, and before bed. That's five minutes right there! Think of it as an investment. Even this small contribution to your mantra practice not only will give you immediate health benefits, it will also bring you great returns of mental, physical, and spiritual equanimity in the long term. Gradually, you will create a life with greater peace and joy through a more dedicated daily practice.

DON'T WORRY

When you're starting a mantra practice, it's easy to become overwhelmed by questions and anxieties. Am I chanting this right? Am I pronouncing the words correctly? At the end of the day, what is most important when it comes to chanting a mantra is the sincerity with which you practice. If you're dedicated to practicing your mantra meditation, the very act of chanting these sacred sounds will be enough to change you. Once you feel more settled into the routine of your practice, try to pair an intention with your mantra, as this will give deeper meaning to your mantra practice.

ADJUST YOUR EXPECTATIONS

People often embark on a meditation journey expecting it to look or feel a certain way. They quickly become attached to a specific, desired outcome. Although it is important to practice with intention, it is also important to be open to whatever occurs. You might feel ecstasy and bliss every time you sit down to meditate. You might even experience emotional upheaval—mantras are designed to shift old patterns, and often that is exactly what they will do. The value of this practice is that it actually takes the mind's tendency to want to be active and uses the mantra as its channel; old destructive thought patterns are broken and new constructive, positive thought patterns are created. This results in a vibrational shift in thought, which translates into a biochemical shift in the body. We each bring our own singular psychology and physiology to the practice. It's important to receive every experience of your practice as valid.

Once you have established the basics of your practice, keep in mind that a variety of elements—sound, intention, meaning, devotion, rhythm, and speed—will make your mantra meditation more effective if you know how to focus on them properly. When you are ready, begin to deepen your practice by exploring these additional elements.

SOUND

The simplest and most basic way to enhance a mantra practice is to focus on the sound of your own chanting. As I have explored through this book, mantra meditation has many benefits, including overriding thought patterns that have a harmful effect on our psychology and physiology. Everyone has maladaptive or ruminative thought patterns; by chanting, we can break up this unconscious dialogue. On a more profound level, the sounds themselves connect us to our true nature by attuning us to primordial vibrations.

INTENTION

It is helpful to establish an intention or goal for your chanting practice once you feel comfortable in your meditation practice. In Sanskrit, this is known as a *sankalpa*, which is an intention that balances the desires of the soul with the practicality of human needs. It is generally a short, positive affirmation that focuses on a specific goal to work toward, such as "I will honor my body," or "I will uphold truthfulness in my life," or "I will be compassionate toward myself and others." It can be called upon to reinforce your true beliefs and guide the choices you make in life.

MEANING

A mantra practice will be more rewarding if you delve into the meaning behind the sound that you are chanting. While the meanings of mantras vary, they are generally connected with a character or quality that you can access within yourself—for example, Aim (pronounced *ayeem*) is related to wisdom and knowledge. If you bring this quality to mind along with your sound and intention for practicing, it will bolster your awareness. In other words, when chanting Aim, you're thinking not only of the wisdom and knowledge that you would like to access within yourself but also of the intention to apply it in your life to achieve a certain outcome. If you simply chant, you will still get benefits, of course—the sounds alone will allow you to transcend your mind. But adding meaning to it will bring you into more substantial relationship with your practice and you will have more effective results.

DEVOTION

As you may recall from chapter 7, love and devotion are the essential feelings that energize the bhakti yoga practice. This creates the awareness of life as an expression of one underlying reality and encourages a shift in attention from the desires of the individual ego to the intelligence of universal consciousness. This practice also encourages connecting to feeling over distant analysis. Devotion will bring grace and ease to your mantra practice, which will, in turn, allow you to be more accepting of the inevitable challenges in life.

RHYTHM

Repetitive activity has a powerful effect on both body and brain. Rhythmic formulas such as mantras help maintain the body's own cardiovascular rhythms. In fact, a 2001 study, funded by the NIH and conducted by researchers at the University of Pavia in Italy, found that repeating yoga mantras slowed respiration and increased variability in cardiovascular rhythms, which indicates better heart health and emotional resilience. As was found in the HeartMath studies, emotions first register physiologically and are then interpreted by the brain; by improving our heart rate variability with mantras, we are also gaining control over our emotional lives. It does this by slowing down breathing and heart rate and modifying baroreflex sensitivity, which is the part of your brain that regulates your blood pressure. The rhythmic actions of chanting mantras can also help to direct the mind into the highest vibratory frequency, merging individual consciousness with universal consciousness.

SPEED

The slower the recitation of a mantra, the greater its power. The silence between the repetition of the mantras is as important as the mantra itself. The sacred sound of the mantra gently leads us back to our silent true nature. There may be certain times, of course, when you have to change the speed of your chanting depending on how you're feeling or how much time you have. If you're tired and drowsy, for example, you may need a faster repetition to keep you alert and engaged. But, typically, your chanting should be slow and methodical.

MANTRAS FOR EVERYDAY LIFE

As I've mentioned before, sacred chants can be found throughout the world and throughout different spiritual and religious traditions. But the ancient Vedic tradition has gone a step further, exploring and refining the use of mantra over thousands of years. I've included the chakra mantra here once again for easy reference, followed by ten Sanskrit mantras from the Vedas that I think are elementary enough, but also beneficial enough, to serve as a good starting point for your practice. While many of those mantras are directed at specific deities, they're actually intended to arouse the qualities related to each deity within you, too.

There is no right or wrong mantra. Ultimately, you should pick the one or ones that appeal most to you and that seem suitable to your current needs in life. You can benefit from any of these mantras—the ultimate goal of all of them is to draw forth your divine nature.

I recommend chanting these for twenty to thirty minutes a day as a starting point. Some people report feeling an improvement immediately, some notice a more gradual effect over several months. Over the course of a routine practice, you should feel greater ease and balance. You may notice that you're not as exhausted at the end of the day or as quick to snap at your partner or kids in the morning in the hectic rush to get everyone to work or school. You'll feel more present and peaceful—and you'll find these effects can ricochet outward, affecting other areas of your life.

AMMA'S CHAKRA MANTRA
(for balancing all of the chakras):

Hari Om,
Nam Lam,
Mam Vam,
Sim Ram,
Vam Yam,
Yam Ham,
Shiva Om,
Swaha

OM (OR AUM) MANTRA

The word, or primordial sound, Om/Aum in the Vedas—which is correlative to Amen in Christianity, Hum in Tibetan, and Amin in Islam—is also sometimes referred to as the word of God. This mantra is the most basic of all mantras, yet it's the most important one: It is the source of all other mantras and is believed to contain all vibratory sounds. This all-encompassing sound of creation is found in the beginning of nearly all mantras.

This mantra is associated with three main energy centers in the body and the three main gods in Hinduism, who represent these energies.

A—is associated with Brahma, the god who embodies the vibration of universal creative energy found in the second, or sacral, chakra.

U—is associated with Lord Vishnu, the god who embodies the sustaining universal force found in the fourth, or heart, chakra.

M—is associated with Lord Shiva, the god who embodies the underlying, unseen principle of consciousness found in the sixth chakra.

Some of the benefits of chanting Om include improving the production of endorphins, making you feel relaxed and refreshed; positive effects in heart health by lowering blood pressure and improving the immune functioning of all the cells in the body; relaxing and rejuvenating the mind, thereby increasing concentration and memory and your ability to learn; and eliminating negative repetitive thoughts as well as helping to decrease stress and promote social connections.

GANESHA MANTRA

Ganesha is the elephant-faced god, who represents the overcoming of obstacles as well as the virtues of focus, self-control, strength, wisdom, and fortitude.

Ganesha, one of the most important gods in Hindu mythology, is said to have been molded from the earth by Parvati, wife of Lord Shiva. When Shiva returned—after being away on a meditative wandering—he found a young boy blocking the doorway. The boy refused to let him in. A battle ensued, and Shiva beheaded Ganesha. When Parvati found Ganesha dead, she became hysterical and threatened to destroy everything. Repentant, Shiva ordered a new head to be found for the boy. The first animal that was available was an elephant—the gods took this and, before breathing life back into his body, offered this to the boy. So Ganesha took on the head of an elephant and the body of a boy, thus becoming one of the most distinctive Hindu gods. As a form of apology, Lord Shiva appointed Ganesha the leader of the Ganas (a Sanskrit word for "group"), which included Shiva's army as well as all the elemental spirits, celestial gods, and all other human and animal forces in nature. Since all of these beings contribute to human success or failure, it is said that by honoring their leader, Ganesha, you honor them all.

This mantra is Om Gam Ganapataye Namah (pronounced *Om gung Gah-nah-pa-tha-yaa namaha*). The literal meaning of this is "Lord Ganapathi, I surrender to you" or "Lord Ganapathi, I offer my deepest salutations to you." This mantra, which corresponds to the first chakra, is beneficial for issues such as fear and anxiety. It also unblocks energy in your physical and energetic bodies, resulting in reduction of pain anywhere in the body, but especially pain located around the base of the spine; makes the mind more stable and balanced; improves focus;

boosts confidence; and assists you when you're undertaking any project or when any problem arises, particularly problems you can see no way through. The Ganesha mantra also bolsters all other mantras by providing a stable base, helping you achieve quicker positive results from the mantra.

SARASWATI MANTRA

Saraswati is the goddess who embodies knowledge, wisdom, discrimination, and the arts. Her name comes from two words, *Saras*, which means river, and *vathi*, meaning related to speech. Saraswati is typically seen wearing a white sari and has four arms, two in the front to symbolize her presence and work in the physical world, and her two back arms to represent her existence and activity in the spiritual realm. She is symbolic of the river of consciousness that organizes, enlivens, and creates wisdom in the world. This mantra is thought to improve memory, speech, and concentration. She also holds a veena, an instrument used to help singers to stay in tune that is believed to have brought all of the Vedic mantras into existence.

Every year, on the fifth day of spring, an Indian celebration dedicated to the worship of the goddess Saraswati called Vasant Panchami occurs. For this, children and college students bring their books and pens to the Saraswati puja—a ceremony held to invoke gods or goddesses—in order to receive her blessings for the school year ahead.

This mantra is Om Aim Namaha (pronounced *Om ayeem namaha*). The literal meaning is "Goddess Saraswati, I surrender to you" or "Goddess Saraswati, I offer my deepest salutations to you." This mantra relates to three chakras: the second (sacral) chakra, the fifth (throat) chakra, and the sixth (third eye) chakra. Given these connections, this mantra connects to the universal source of wisdom and knowledge, increases intelligence, supports and helps develop the power of voice and speech, and enhances the ability to concentrate—and is especially useful with conditions like attention deficit–hyperactivity disorder (ADHD).

LAKSHMI MANTRA

Lakshmi literally translates to "goal." As such, this goddess is also typically depicted with four arms, though hers symbolize the four aims of life: dharma (virtuous living in accord with one's worldly and spiritual duties), artha (living a purposeful life), kama (noble desires that support a meaningful life), and moksha (liberation from the cycle of birth and death). She is sometimes seen as part of a trinity with Saraswati and Durga. Lakshmi is the embodiment of all divine feminine virtues: prosperity, abundance, good fortune, beauty, and health. These chants will bring all of those energies flowing into your life.

There is a story known as Sagara Manthan, or the churning of the ocean of milk. In this story, Amaravati, the kingdom of the god Indra, became cursed and as a result was taken over by demons. A beleaguered Indra banded together with other gods and sought help from Lord Vishnu, who advised him to churn the ocean of milk and seek the divine nectar of immortality, called amrit, which would help them to regain the kingdom.

The churning brought forth many things from the ocean, including halahala (poison), which Lord Shiva—the healer of sickness and remover of poisons—drank and kept in his throat in order to save all of creation; Goddess Lakshmi also emerged from the churning milk, and, finally, Dhanvantri (the god of healing) rose from it, too, holding the pot of amrit in his hands. The gods received the divine nectar to restore their powers.

This story, as with all Hindu stories, is rich in symbolism. The ocean of milk represents the mind as the residing place for both gods and demons. As you begin to churn your mind to purify it, the first thing to be released is poison—all the toxic qualities and thoughts that keep us from knowing our own highest Self. The gods represent our inherently pure qualities, such as dharma (virtuous, responsible activities), happiness, joy, intelligence, and compassion. The demons represent our inherently negative qualities, such as impure thoughts and emotions that lead to suffering, including greed, anger, and jealousy. Knowing that these two extremes exist within each of us is key to making progress on a spiritual path. You must acknowledge—and balance—all of the positive and negative qualities that commingle within us in order to deliver the treasures of human life.

Lakshmi herself symbolizes material wealth and abundance. She showered the gods with blessings at seeing their humility as well as their struggle to repent. Thus, it is believed, when you realize your misdeeds and work toward correcting them, keeping the ego in check, Lakshmi will return prosperity to your life.

This mantra is Om Srim Namaha (pronounced *Om Shreem Namaha*). The literal translation is "Goddess Lakshmi, I surrender to you" or "Goddess Lakshmi, I offer my deepest salutations to you." Lakshmi is the source of all wealth, so this mantra will connect you to that vibration of abundance. It will also purify your mind and help to keep you focused on pure thoughts and toward spirituality. This mantra also represents the heart chakra and, as such, helps to connect you to your heart's desires. Additionally, it is believed to increase vigor and vitality, to help to get you on track with your life's purpose, increase physical beauty, and awaken inner joy.

DURGA MANTRA

Durga, which literally means "invincible," is the name of the warrior goddess whose mythology represents freedom from evils; she is the mother goddess who will unleash her anger against wrongdoing or threat to peace. She is also considered the highest form of divine feminine power, or Shakti. Durga is worshipped for her ferocious spirit as much as for her gracious nature.

Her origin is recounted in the story of an immortal demon named Mahishasura, who could change his outer form but never his inner evil and took over the heavens and earth. When the gods could not defeat him, they decided to combine their essences to create the goddess Durga. Each one gave her their weapons and she single-handedly destroyed Mahishasura as well as all of his armies.

Her mantra is Om Krim Namaha (pronounced *Om Kreem Namaha*). The literal translation is "Goddess Durga, I surrender to you" or "Goddess Durga, I offer my deepest salutations to you." As Durga is associated with the third (solar plexus) chakra, which is connected with our digestive organs, liver, gallbladder, pancreas, stomach, spleen, and our willpower, this mantra will enliven the organs of digestion, help to overcome our negative tendencies as well as face negativity in the world around us, decrease depression, bestow courage, and increase willpower and strength in life.

NARAYANI MANTRA

Narayani is the combined form of three goddesses—Saraswati, Lakshmi, and Durga. Narayani is the supreme form of the divine mother, or the Great Goddess. (Amma is, as I mentioned earlier, considered to be the first documented human incarnation of Narayani.) Narayani represents feminine power and is the ultimate form of Shakti, or primordial, divine feminine strength. Narayani is worshipped as the energy behind this universe and, therefore, as the one who holds the power to elevate consciousness so the unity with the divine can be achieved.

There was a time in history when there was balance between male and female energies in the world, considered the Golden Ages. Our current time, however, has an imbalance of these energies, with a greater dominance of male energy. The Narayani mantra helps to remedy this energetic imbalance and raise the divine feminine energy within us all.

This mantra is Om Namo Narayani (pronounced *Om namo NaaraayanE*). This is the strongest Shakti mantra (divine feminine energy) and enlivens this energy in the person chanting the mantra—this benefits men and women, since Shakti is seen as the creative force in all of life. In chanting this mantra, it will help the person surrender to divine will and includes all of the benefits of chanting the Saraswati, Lakshmi, and Durga mantras combined.

GAYATRI MANTRA

Gayatri is the goddess who is considered the mother of the Vedas, the ancient scriptures of India. She is a protector, a goddess of wisdom, and one who confers enlightenment. The Gayatri mantra is one of the oldest and most sacred Vedic mantras. This mantra was given to the world as a great blessing to the Vishvamitra, an eminent king, who, when passing through the forest with his troops, was vanquished after attempting to fight the great sage Vasishtha.

After his defeat, Vishvamitra renounced everything and went into the forest alone to enter into a deep meditation. After many years, he eventually was blessed as a great sage for conquering his vices of anger, lust, greed, attachment, arrogance, and jealousy. This blessing that flowed to Vishvamitra as merit for his spiritual accomplishment is now known as the Gayatri mantra.

Gayatri is represented by five goddesses in one and is typically depicted as having five heads. Each head represents a prana, the vital energies that flow through you, enlivening the body and mind.

This mantra is Om bhur bhuva swaha; Tat savitur ver-aanyam; Bhargo devasya dheemahi; Dheeyoyo nah pracho-dayaat (pronounced *Om bhoor bhu-wah swa-ha; tat savi-tur vareen-yam; bhar-go de-va-sya dheem-a-hi; dhiyo yo nah pra-cho-day-at*). The literal meaning of this is "Oh, mother, you en-compass the earth, space, and celestial realms beyond. You are that [aspect of the divine that is beyond words] most beloved goddess of the sun. We meditate on your all purifying divine effulgence. May you enlighten our intelligence." The primary benefit of this mantra is that it promotes healing by balancing all five of our pranas.

The first of these—also named prana—energizes all the other pranas. It's associated with the heart chakra and the third eye; when it's blocked, the heart or lungs will become disturbed or diseased. This block can also show up as fear, anxiety, and depression, and can lead to asthma, stroke, poor concentration, and general dullness. The second is udana, which corresponds to the throat chakra. It supports blood flow to the brain. It also controls speech, voice, and the expression of thoughts. Poor flow of udana will show up as tonsillitis, throat issues, thyroid issues, difficulties in thinking clearly or being able to express oneself, weight loss, speech problems, and a lack of efficiency in physical or mental work. Third, there is samana, seated in the solar plexus or third chakra; this fuels the digestive organs and balances and stabilizes all other pranas. This energy also keeps the ego in check, maintains harmony within ourselves, and supports mental peace. When out of balance, this will show up as agitation, poor digestion of food, ulcers, lethargy, and anger. The fourth is apana, which is related to the first and second chakras. This energy is responsible for getting rid of the body's waste matter. It's also responsible for the reproductive organs and helps to eliminate toxic thoughts and feelings. Indications that apana is out of balance could be emotional struggles, diarrhea, constipation, menstrual issues, and sexual problems. The last one is vyana, which is the energy that can be found throughout our entire body, running through every one of the subtle energy channels. It governs the movement of prana throughout the body. It dictates the flow of blood and lymphatic fluid in the body and the flow of thoughts in the mind. Imbalances will show up as edema, poor circulation, neuropathy, multiple sclerosis, lack of coordination, and erratic thoughts.

VISHNU MANTRA

Lord Vishnu is the embodiment of both the supporting force in the universe and of dharma (righteous living). Lord Vishnu had nine earthly incarnations at nine different times when dharma was in decline. Each avatar took a different form, ranging from a half lion/half man named Narasimha to a naughty, magical, wise boy named Krishna. Each time Lord Vishnu came to teach a different lesson to humankind out of his love and compassion for the human race. So it will come as no surprise he is associated with the heart chakra.

This mantra is Om Namo Narayanaya (pronounced *Om namo Narayanaya*). Narayana is another name for Lord Vishnu, which has multiple translations, such as "Supreme being" and "One who rests in waters." The literal translation is "Narayana, I surrender to you" or "Narayana, I offer my deepest salutations to you."

This mantra is described in the Narayana Upanishad: "Verily, one who contemplates on this eight-syllabled chant attains good health all his life. He enjoys prosperity fit for a king, knowledge, and status of a ruler. He attains immortality." It is also believed to confer prosperity, love, power, abundance, and glory; improve skills as an administrator and leader; increase wisdom; reduce egoism; and relax the nervous system.

SHIVA MANTRA

Lord Shiva, one of the three main gods in Hinduism, is the source of all consciousness. He destroys ignorance within us and throughout the world. He is a four-armed deity with dreadlocks dancing in the middle of a circle of flames with his feet on a dwarf. The story that accompanies this being is as rich as this illustration and conveys a deep spiritual truth.

The dwarf depicted is Apasmara, who represents the ignorance of the ego. The ego cannot be killed because it would undermine each individual's personal journey to suppress the ego

through spirituality. As a result, Apasmara was immortal—
and took great pleasure in torturing those who prayed to Shiva.
Finally, his arrogance grew so strong that he challenged Shiva
to a battle. Lord Shiva performed the tandava, a cosmic dance
representing the divine flow of consciousness. During this
dance, Shiva brought the diabolical Apasmara into submission
with his foot. The statue of Lord Shiva symbolizes the need to
persevere in suppressing the ego through constant effort, and
not be lazy in the process of realizing the highest goals of yoga.
Shiva, as the universal consciousness, is the only reality that
can keep the ego in submission.

This mantra is Om Namah Shivaya (pronounced *Om Namah
Shiviiya*). This is part of Amma's chakra mantra offered earlier
in the book. This powerful chant connects us to all five elements
and harmonizes all the chakras in the body, bringing balance
to the entire body and mind. It also helps with depression and
insomnia; increases mental stability and calmness; and dissolves
the ego.

DHANVANTRI MANTRA

Dhanvantri is an incarnation of Lord Vishnu, the father of
Ayurvedic medicine. He also happened to be one of the Siddhas.
So he brought Ayurveda as a form of medicine that could be
practiced by the majority of people, but he also knew of the secrets of Siddha medicine, reserved for the select few. Dhanvantri,
then, is considered the source of health and balance and grants
long life and even immortality. It was Dhanvantri who trained

the Sushruta sages, the first surgeons. He has the power to prevent disease and resolve incurable conditions.

This mantra is Om Shri Dhanvantre Namah (pronounced *Om shree Dhanvantrayaa namaha*). This is one of the principal Sanskrit healing mantras. This can also be recited to help prevent sickness or assist in healing those who are sick.

Having practiced mantra for much of my life, I've come to learn that what I've truly been in pursuit of is silence as the goal of sacred sound. This is what all sound eventually pools down to, after all. It is through the power and vibration of sound—in the reciting of my bija mantra in my mind—that I came to the deepest reservoir of stillness and peace. There are many words for silence in Sanskrit—two of the most significant ones are *maun* and *nis-sabda*. *Maun* means silence as we generally understand it—quietness and stillness. But *nis-sabda* means "that which is not sound"—beyond body, mind, and creation. It means, in essence, transcending sound. This is a place of peace and bliss, and its only intention is the expression of universal love. It is from this place that we are able to tap into our natural ability to heal, by creating a connection to our true selves—which is also a place of oneness with the universal energy of life.

ACKNOWLEDGMENTS

I am deeply honored to have been selected to peer into the sacred chambers of the Siddhas; I thank them for their enduring love and compassion for humankind, which have silently shaped the history of the world. I also want to thank my beautiful husband, Joshua, who lives in constant reverberation of love and devotion to life itself. Through his example, he has taught me the power of mantra and devotion. And I wouldn't have been introduced to the mantras had it not been for my mother's fascination with the science of spirituality. I am blessed to have had such a unique and dynamic woman teach me to have the curiosity to look beneath the veil of nature. I also want to thank my agent, Heather Jackson, not only for her ongoing professional support and encouragement but also for the degree of heart and perseverance she has invested in bringing this ancient knowledge to the world. I also want to extend my heartfelt gratitude to Nell Casey, my writer. Her contribution to the book was immense and her intellectual reframing of the esoteric concepts of Vedic knowledge and the Siddhas helped bring this ancient knowledge to a modern audience. I want to extend my deep appreciation to Dr. David Muehsam from the National Institute of Biostructures and Biosystems in Italy and the Consciousness and Healing Initiative in the United States. David's academic generosity in sharing relevant research in the field of sound medicine was critical to the scientific foundation for many of the concepts in this book. David is as bighearted as he is brilliant. This book grew out of an earlier collaboration with chanting researcher and practitioner Gemma Perry, who provided scientific input into how sound and music affect people from around the world. She shared her ideas, research, and understanding of global chanting traditions, yoga philosophy, and the psychological and physiological effects of mantra meditation. I am grateful to Gemma for her contributions.

APPENDIX: MANTRA Q&A

My patients have many questions for me when they begin their mantra meditations. And understandably so. It is natural to feel uncertain at first. In this appendix, I have answered some of the most commonly asked questions by my patients so that you may refer to this as a guide in the early days of setting up your practice.

Do I always have to practice mantra in my sacred space?

After they've sustained a routine mantra meditation practice for a few months, my patients feel as if it is stored in their hearts and minds. This does not simply mean they've memorized their mantras; it also means the feeling they associate with meditation has become a kind of sense memory. Once this has occurred, you can practice your mantra anytime, anywhere: in the car, at the grocery store, standing on the subway. My husband chants his mantra while he's doing his physical yoga practice. He simply repeats the mantra with each position. In doing this, he brings an even more mindful focus to his asanas by using the mantra to concentrate his attention on the sensation of his muscles contracting and relaxing and aligning with his breath. Having said all this, it is still ideal to try to take some time in the day, if possible, to practice in a quiet place with your eyes closed. When you

practice consistently in one place, you will imbue it with the
energy of your mantra.

Will my child benefit from learning a mantra?

Absolutely! Mantras are terrific tools for kids. They can
help them to develop a healthy sense of self and cultivate an
early sense of spiritual connection. Multiple studies have
shown that children who learn mantra meditation are able
to allay anxiety, improve focus and concentration, and reduce symptoms of ADHD. One of the best ways to introduce young kids to mantra is through singing. I particularly
like the Saraswati mantra, Om Aim Namaha. This is often
chanted by young students in India to relax and help them
do well on exams. I even chant this with my son sometimes when he's having trouble with his homework. For
very young children, I suggest introducing them simply to
Om. You can encourage them to play with the tone, speed,
and volume. If they don't seem interested, that's fine. You
can always reintroduce the idea of a mantra practice later.
The good news is that even if they aren't practicing, they
can benefit from you chanting around them, whether out
loud or silently.

**If someone is recovering from an illness, such as a stroke,
can they still benefit?**

Yes. A person doesn't even have to chant to see positive
results. Research has shown that simply listening to someone
else perform a mantra practice is an effective way to benefit
from the sacred sounds. This is what happens during the

puja when we listen to Amma and others chant. You can sit by your family member's side and chant, or play a recorded mantra for him. It's beneficial to have mantras playing in the background while you're engaged in another activity—such as driving or cooking—as well.

Do pets respond to mantra?

Yes, especially if your pets are anxious or traumatized or if you have an animal that suffers from separation anxiety. Obviously, our pets aren't going to chant along with us, but they can benefit from listening. Mantras create a zone of comfort, safety, and love that our beloved pets soak up, whether they're coming from an owner's voice or from a CD. There's no one mantra that is more effective than others for animals—ultimately, as is true with humans, it comes down to what your pet responds to instinctually. If your animal leaves the room or otherwise seems disinterested during the mantra practice, that's a good indicator that they're not feeling it. Many of my patients, however, report that their pets spontaneously gravitate toward them while they are chanting.

What's the best time of day to do my mantra meditation? Are there times when I shouldn't do it?

There is never a time of day when you cannot do a mantra practice, but there *are* times of day that are considered to be the most beneficial. These times correlate to the vata hours between 2 and 6 a.m. and 2 and 6 p.m. The morning hours are when the mind tends to be the most alert, and therefore people typically experience the most clarity and focus during their practice; the hours in the evening tend to be when the body experiences a lull in energy and a mantra practice helps to revive the mind and body. I would also caution that there are certain stimulating mantras—such as the mantras used to balance the kapha dosha (offered in chapter 6)—that shouldn't be chanted before bedtime, as they may interfere with your sleep.

Can my partner and I do mantra meditation together, or is there a potential for conflict?

Doing a mantra meditation with your partner or family is an amazing experience and highly recommended. This allows you to build intimacy and grow together. Studies show that when people meditate together, their brain waves show greater coherence with one another. There is the potential for far more conflict when people grow apart by *not* sharing their interests, including their meditation practices. When you do it as a couple or a family, you can share experiences and insights as well as physical shifts that may occur outside your practice.

If I'm using a mantra from another culture or religion, does that mean that I am practicing that religion?

Mantras are seen as universal sounds and not specific to any particular religion. Even though religious groups have adopted certain mantras, they are considered a secular and scientific practice with mental, physical, and spiritual benefits. While they do require emotion and sincerity to activate properly, they need not have any religious connotation to be effective. Because mantras are considered to transcend the mind, they are tools for universal benefit.

What if I already have a Transcendental Meditation mantra practice?

If you have already been given a mantra through a particular lineage, the recommendation is to not switch from one mantra to another. Mantras are passed on through a spiritual lineage in order to activate them. It is important to respect this by not shifting to another mantra. There are, however, specific Vedic celebrations—for example, special occasions when Hindu deities are honored—when everyone is invited to chant particular mantras in celebration. For a daily practice, however, it is best to consistently chant the original mantra given to you.

NOTES

CHAPTER 2: THE BIOLOGY OF SOUND

1. Anthony J. DeCasper and Melanie J. Spence, "Prenatal Maternal Speech Influences Newborns' Perception of Speech Sounds," *Infant Behavior and Development*, no. 9 (1986): 1.
2. Jessica Timmons (medically reviewed by Debra Sullivan, Ph.D., MSN, RN, CNE, COI), "When Can a Fetus Hear?," *Healthline*, https://www.healthline.com/health/pregnancy/when-can-a-fetus -hear#1.
3. DeCasper and Spence, "Prenatal Maternal Speech," 1.
4. Tim Urban, "Everything You Should Know About Sound," *Wait But Why*, March 6, 2016, https://waitbutwhy.com/2016/03/sound.html.
5. Ingo R. Titze, *Principles of Voice Production* (Upper Saddle River, NJ: Prentice Hall, 1994), 188.
6. Urban, "Everything You Should Know About Sound."
7. S. Puria and J. J. Rosowski, "Békésy's Contribution to Our Present Understanding of Sound Conduction to the Inner Ear," *Hearing Research*, no. 293 (2012): 21.
8. Tanya Lewis, "5 Fascinating Facts About Fetal Ultrasounds," *Live Science*, May 16, 2013, https://www.livescience.com/32071-history-of -fetal-ultrasound.html.
9. "Ultrasonic Sound," Hyperphysics, http://hyperphysics.phy-astr.gsu .edu/hbase/Sound/usound.html#c1.
10. Christian Nordqvist, "How Do Ultrasound Scans Work?," *Medical News Today*, https://www.medicalnewstoday.com/articles/245491 .php.
11. David Schlesinger et al., "MR-Guided Focused Ultrasound Surgery, Present and Future," *Medical Physics*, no. 40 (2013): 8.
12. Anne Roberts, M.D., "Magnetic Resonance-Guided Focused Ultra- sound for Uterine Fibroids," *Seminars in Interventional Radiology*, no. 25 (2008): 394–405.

13. "Uterine Fibroids," Focused Ultrasound Foundation, https://www .fusfoundation.org/diseases-and-conditions/womens-health/uterine -fibroids.

14. M. J. Schnabel et al., "Shock Wave Lithotripsy in Germany," *Urologe A*, no. 54 (2015): 9.

15. P. P. Dobrakowski et al., "MR-Guided Focused Ultrasound: A New Generation of Treatment of Parkinson's Disease, Essential Tremor and Neuropathic Pain," *Interventional Neuroradiology*, no. 20 (2014): 275–82.

16. "Essential Tremor," Focused Ultrasound Foundation, https://www.fus foundation.org/diseases-and-conditions/neurological/essential-tremor.

17. Daniel Coluccia et al., "First Noninvasive Thermal Ablation of a Brain Tumor with MR-Guided Focused Ultrasound," *Journal of Therapeutic Ultrasound*, no. 2 (2014): 17; and S. A. Quadri et al., "High-Intensity Focused Ultrasound: Past, Present, and Future in Neurosurgery," *Neurosurgical Focus* (2018).

18. Nicole Cobler, "Less-Invasive Prostate Treatment Receives FDA Clearance," *Statesman*, https://www.statesman.com/NEWS/20180705 /Less-invasive-prostate-cancer-treatment-receives-FDA-clearance.

19. Charles Bankhead, "'Cautious Optimism' for HIFU in Prostate Cancer," *MedPageToday*, May 13, 2016, https://www.medpagetoday .com/MeetingCoverage/AUA/57896.

20. K. L. Lee et al., "The Primary Cilium Functions as a Mechanical and Calcium Signaling Nexus," *Cilia Journal*, no. 4 (2015).

21. David A. Hoey, Matthew E. Downs, and Christopher R. Jacobs, "The Mechanics of the Primary Cilium: An Intricate Structure with Complex Function," *Journal of Biomechanics*, no. 45 (2012): 17–26.

22. Thierry Steiner, Ph.D., "The Biology of Fear- and Anxiety-Related Behaviors," *Dialogues in Clinical Neuroscience*, no. 4 (2002): 231–49.

23. H. Stefan Bracha, M.D., et al., "Postmortem Locus Coeruleus Neuron Count in Three American Veterans with Probable or Possible War-Related PTSD," *Journal of Neuropsychiatry and Clinical Neurosciences*, no. 17 (2005): 503–9.

24. Cassandra D. Gould van Praag et al., "Mind-Wandering and Alteration to Default Mode Network Connectivity When Listening to Naturalistic versus Artificial Sounds," *Scientific Reports*, no. 7 (2017).

25. Stephanie Pappas, "Oxytocin: Facts about the 'Cuddle Hormone,'" *Live Science*, June 4, 2015, https://www.livescience.com/42198-what -is-oxytocin.html.

26. Willis Milham, *Time and Timekeepers* (Detroit, MI: Omnigraphics Inc., 1996).

27. Kevin Knudson, "Pendulum, Pendulum on the Wall: This 'Odd Kind of Sympathy' Syncs Them All," *Forbes*, July 29, 2015, https://www .forbes.com/sites/kevinknudson/2015/07/29/pendulum-pendulum -on-the-wall/#3c3795713fb0.

28. Idan Tal et al., "Neural Entrainment to the Beat: The 'Missing Pulse' Phenomenon," *Journal of Neuroscience*, no. 37 (2017).

29. History of Music Therapy, *American Music Therapy Association*, https://www.musictherapy.org/about/history/.

30. Jenna Spencer, "A Historical Review of Music Therapy and the Department of Veteran Affairs," *Music Therapy Commons*, https://digital commons.molloy.edu/cgi/viewcontent.cgi?article=1011&context=etd.

31. History of Music Therapy, *American Music Therapy Association*.

32. History of Music Therapy, *American Music Therapy Association*.

33. S. Koelsch, T. Fritz, and G. Schlaug, "Amygdala Activity Can Be Modulated by Unexpected Chord Functions during Music Listening," *Neuroreport*, no. 19 (2008).

34. Chakravarthi Kanduri et al., "The Effect of Listening to Music on Human Transcriptome," *PeerJ* (March 12, 2015).

35. Sergio Castillo-Pérez, M.D., et al., "Effects of Music Therapy on Depression Compared with Psychotherapy," *The Arts in Psychotherapy*, no. 37 (2010): 387–90.

36. Marianne J. E. van der Heijden et al., "Do Hospitalized Premature Infants Benefit from Music Interventions: A Systematic Review of Randomized Controlled Trials," *PLOS One*, no. 11 (September 8, 2016).

37. Richard Gray, "Music Can Boost Your Immune System," *Telegraph*, August 16, 2008, https://www.telegraph.co.uk/news/uknews/2569640 /Music-can-boost-your-immune-system.html.

38. J. Bradt, C. Dileo, and N. Potvin, "Music for Stress and Anxiety Reduction in Coronary Heart Disease Patients," *Cochrane Database System Review*, no. 12 (2013).

39. Mitzi Baker, "Music Moves Brain to Pay Attention, Stanford Study Finds," Stanford Medicine News Center, August 1, 2007, https://med

.stanford.edu/news/all-news/2007/07/music-moves-brain-to-pay-attention-stanford-study-finds.html.

40. Michael H. Thaut et al., "Neurologic Music Therapy Improves Executive Function and Emotional Adjustment in Traumatic Brain Injury Rehabilitation," *Annals of the New York Academy of Sciences*, no. 57 (2009): 263–307.

41. Kurt Braunlich et al., "Rhythmic Auditory Cues Shape Neural Network Recruitment in Parkinson's Disease during Repetitive Motor Behavior," *European Journal of Neuroscience* (March 2019): 849–58, https://doi: 10.1111/ejn.14227.

42. "What Is Vibroacoustic Therapy," http://vibroacoustic.blogspot.com/2015/09/history-and-research-of-vibroacoustic.html.

43. Olav Skille, *Manual of Vibroacoustics* (Levanger, Norway: ISVA Publications, 1991).

44. Jeff Hooper, "An Introduction to Vibroacoustic Therapy and an Examination of Its Place in Music Therapy Practice," *British Journal of Music Therapy*, no. 15 (December 1, 2001): 69–77, https://doi.org/10.1177/135945750101500205.

45. "What Is Vibroacoustic Therapy?," *Your Inner Essence*, https://www.yourinneressence.com/news-article.php?id=11.

46. Sophia Roosth, "Screaming Yeast: Sonocytology, Cytoplasmic Milieus, and Cellular Subjectivities," *University of Chicago Press Journals*, no. 35 (2009): 332–50, https://doi.org/10.1086/596646.

47. Andrew E. Pelling, "The Dark Side of the Cell," http://www.darksideofcell.info/bg.html.

CHAPTER 3: SPACE IS NOT EMPTY

1. "On the Principia Mathematica," University of Cambridge Digital Library, https://cudl.lib.cam.ac.uk/view/PR-ADV-B-00039-00001/1.

2. "Newton's Laws of Motion," Glenn Research Center, https://www.grc.nasa.gov/www/k-12/airplane/newton.html.

3. "Vortex Theory," http://descartes.cyberbrahma.com/vortex.html.

4. "The Mechanical Universe," Ideas of Cosmology, https://history.aip.org/exhibits/cosmology/ideas/mechuniverse.htm.

5. "Quantum Theory Timeline," Particle Adventure, http://www.particleadventure.org/other/history/quantumt.html.

6. "The Nobel Prize in Physics 1918," Nobel Prize, https://www.nobelprize.org/prizes/physics/1918/summary/.

7. William Harris and Craig Freudenrich, Ph.D., "How Light Works," How Stuff Works, https://science.howstuffworks.com/light6.htm.

8. Chad Orzel, "Einstein's Complicated Relationship with Quantum Physics," *Forbes*, November 13, 2018, https://www.forbes.com/sites /chadorzel/2018/11/13/einsteins-complicated-relationship-with-quan tum-physics/#4a8abce03504.

9. "History and Quantum Mechanical Quantities," Boundless Physics, https://courses.lumenlearning.com/boundless-physics/chapter /history-and-quantum-mechanical-quantities/.

10. Nola Taylor Redd, "Einstein's Theory of General Relativity," Space .com, November 7, 2017, https://www.space.com/17661-theory-general -relativity.html.

11. Pedro Ferreira, "General Relativity: Einstein's Insight," *New Scientist*, https://www.newscientist.com/article/mg20727671-900-general -relativity-einsteins-insight/.

12. Brian Dodson, "Quantum 'Spooky Action at a Distance' Travels at Least 10,000 Times Faster than Light," *New Atlas*, March 10, 2013, https://newatlas.com/quantum-entanglement-speed-10000-faster -light/26587/.

13. "Einstein Attacks Quantum Theory; Scientist and Two Colleagues Find It Is Not 'Complete' Even Though 'Correct,'" *New York Times*, May 4, 1935, https://www.nytimes.com/1935/05/04/archives/einstein -attacks-quantum-theory-scientist-and-two-colleagues-find.html.

14. "Nonlocality and Entanglement," *Physics of the Universe*, https://www .physicsoftheuniverse.com/topics_quantum_nonlocality.html.

15. Gabriel Popkin, "Einstein's 'Spooky Action at a Distance' Spotted in Objects Almost Big Enough to See," *Science Mag*, April 25, 2018, https://www.sciencemag.org/news/2018/04/einstein-s-spooky-action -distance-spotted-objects-almost-big-enough-see.

16. "Bell's Theorem," *Scholarpedia*, http://www.scholarpedia.org/article /Bell%27s_theorem.

17. Jake Parks, "Quantum Entanglement Loophole Quashed by Quasar Light," *Astronomy.com*, August 23, 2018, http://www.astronomy.com /news/2018/08/distant-quasars-confirm-quantum-entanglement.

18. John Markoff, "Sorry, Einstein. Quantum Study Suggests 'Spooky Action' Is Real," *New York Times*, https://www.nytimes.com/2015/10 /22/science/quantum-theory-experiment-said-to-prove-spooky-inter actions.html.

19. "What Does Brahman Mean?," Yogapedia, https://www.yogapedia .com/definition/5274/brahman.

20. Amy Vaughn, "Brahman, the Tao, and the Ground of Being," *Yoga to Ease Anxiety*, July 9, 2016, http://www.yogatoeaseanxiety.com/blog /brahman-the-tao-and-the-ground-of-being.

21. James G. Lochtefeld, Ph.D., *The Illustrated Encyclopedia of Hinduism* (New York: Rosen Publishing Group, 2002), 433.

22. Albert Einstein and Leopold Infeld, *The Evolution of Physics: From Early Concepts to Relativity and Quanta* (Cambridge, UK: Cambridge University Press, 1938).

23. Philip Ball, "The Strange Link between the Human Mind and Quantum Physics," BBC, February 16, 2017, http://www.bbc.com /earth/story/20170215-the-strange-link-between-the-human-mind -and-quantum-physics.

24. Kelly Neill, "The Most Beautiful Experiment," *The Observer Effect*, https://theobservereffect.wordpress.com/the-most-beautiful-exper iment/.

25. Anil Ananthaswamy, "Closed Loophole Confirms the Unreality of the Quantum World," *Quanta*, July 25, 2018, https://www.quantamagazine .org/closed-loophole-confirms-the-unreality-of-the-quantum-world -20180725/.

26. Ball, "The Strange Link."

27. Ball, "The Strange Link."

28. "Akasha," Eastern Spirituality, https://www.eastern-spirituality.com /glossary/spirituality-terms/a-definitions/akasha.

29. Dylan Campbell, "Aristotle's on the Heavens," *Ancient History Encyclopedia*, October 16, 2016, https://www.ancient.eu/article/959 /aristotles-on-the-heavens/.

30. "René Descartes," *Stanford Encyclopedia of Philosophy*, https://plato .stanford.edu/entries/descartes/.

31. Beverley Rubik, Ph.D., and Harry Jabs, M.S., "Revisiting the Aether in Science," *Cosmos and History: The Journal of Natural and Social Philosophy*, no. 14 (2018): 239–55, https://pdfs.semanticscholar.org /c609/a2bc70e7245a91a0eeb814923f1e67983d0b.pdf.

32. Rubik and Jabs, "Revisiting the Aether in Science," 239–55.

33. Rubik and Jabs, "Revisiting the Aether in Science," 239–55.

34. P. W. Milonni and M. L. Shih, "Zero Point Energy in Early Quantum Theory," *American Journal of Physics*, no. 8 (1991): 684–98.

35. Charles Choi, "In the Beginning," PBS, June 13, 2012, https://www.pbs.org/wgbh/nova/article/in-the-beginning/.

36. Gordon Kane, "Are Virtual Particles Really Constantly Popping in and out of Existence? Or Are They Merely a Mathematical Bookkeeping Device for Quantum Mechanics?," *Scientific American*, October 9, 2006, https://www.scientificamerican.com/article/are-virtual-particles-rea/.

37. "Zero-Point Energy," *Encyclopedia Britannica*, https://www.britannica.com/science/zero-point-energy.

38. Peter Baksa, "The Zero Point Field: How Thoughts Become Matter?," *Huffington Post*, https://www.huffpost.com/entry/zero-point-field_n_913831?ec_carp=1915546673184137575.

39. Lynne McTaggart, *The Field: The Quest for the Secret Force of the Universe* (New York: HarperCollins, 2002).

40. Eastwood, "What Is Everything? The Nature of the Universe & Human Consciousness: What Matter & Mind Are Made Of," *Mind over Matter*, November 24, 2018, https://www.mindovermatterpower.com/2018/11/24/what-is-everything-the-nature-of-the-universe-human-consciousness-what-matter-mind-are-made-of-fields-zpf/.

41. McTaggart, *The Field*.

CHAPTER 4: THE HUMAN BIOFIELD

1. "The Three Doshas: The Keys to Your Individual Nature," *Eat Taste Heal*, http://www.eattasteheal.com/ayurveda101/eth_bodytypes.htm.

2. "Field, Physics," *Encyclopedia Britannica*, https://www.britannica.com/science/field-physics.

3. Jim Lucas, "What Is the Strong Force?," *Live Science*, November 1, 2014, https://www.livescience.com/48575-strong-force.html.

4. "Science of the Heart: Exploring the Role of the Heart in Human Performance," HeartMath Institute, https://www.heartmath.org/research/science-of-the-heart/energetic-communication/.

5. "Willem Einthoven and the Electrocardiogram," *Past Medical History*, May 9, 2017, https://www.pastmedicalhistory.co.uk/willem-einthoven-and-the-electrocardiogram/.

6. L. F. Haas, "Hans Berger (1873–1941), Richard Caton (1842–1926), and Electroencephalography," *Journal of Neurology, Neurosurgery & Psychiatry*, no. 74 (2003), http://dx.doi.org/10.1136/jnnp.74.1.9.

7. Haas, "Hans Berger."

8. Haas, "Hans Berger."

9. Paul Weiss, "Perspectives in the Field of Morphogenesis," *Quarterly Review of Biology*, vol. 25, no. 2 (1950): 177–98, https://www.jstor.org/stable/i330312

10. Beverly Rubik, Ph.D., "The Biofield: Bridge Between Mind and Body," *Cosmos and History: The Journal of Natural and Social Philosophy*, 11 (2015): 83–96.

11. Rubik, "The Biofield," 83–96.

12. Rubik, "The Biofield," 83–96.

13. Mary Jo Kreitzer, Ph.D., RN, FAAN, and Rob Saper, MD, MPH, "Exploring the Biofield," *Global Advances in Health and Medicine*, no. 4 (2015), https://www.ncbi.nlm.nih.gov/pmc/articles/PMC4654790/.

14. Rubik, "The Biofield," 83–96.

15. Patrick Olivelle, *The Early Upanishads* (Oxford, UK: Oxford University Press, 2014), 12–14.

16. "Pancha Kosha," Yogapedia, https://www.yogapedia.com/definition/6901/pancha-kosha.

17. "Nadi," Yogapedia, https://www.yogapedia.com/definition/5028/nadi.

18. Shamini Jain, Ph.D., Jennifer Daubinmier, Ph.D., and Deepak Chopra, MD, FACP, "Indo-Tibetan Philosophical and Medical Systems: Perspectives on the Biofield," *Global Advances in Health and Medicine* (2015): 16–24, https://www.ncbi.nlm.nih.gov/pmc/articles/PMC4654787/.

19. William Shakespeare, *As You Like It* (Mineola, NY: Dover Thrift Editions, 1998).

20. "Jacques Benveniste," *Encyclopedia Britannica*, https://www.britannica.com/biography/Jacques-Benveniste.

21. Daniel J. Benor, *Consciousness, Bioenergy, and Healing: Self-Healing and Energy Medicine for the 21st Century* (Medford, NJ: Wholistic Healing Publications, 2004), 266.

22. John Maddox, James Randi, and Walter W. Stewart, "High-Dilution Experiments a Delusion," *Nature* (July 28, 1988): 287–90.

23. Jacques Benveniste, "Dr. Jacques Benveniste Replies," *Nature* (1988): 291.

24. E. Davenas et al., "Human Basophil Degranulation Triggered by Very Dilute Antiserum against IgE," *Nature* (1988): 816–18.

25. Francis Beauvais, *Ghosts of Molecules: The Case of the "Memory of Water"* (Collection Mille-Mondes, 2016).

26. Artem Cherkasov et al., "QSAR Modeling: Where Have You Been? Where Are You Going To?" *Journal of Medicinal Chemistry*, no. 57 (2014): 4977–5010, doi: 10.1021/jm4004285.

27. Y. Thomas, "The History of the Memory of Water," *Homeopathy*, no. 96 (2007): 151–57, https://www.ncbi.nlm.nih.gov/pubmed/17678810.

28. McTaggart, *The Field*, 68.

29. Beverly Rubik, A. J. Brooks, and G. E. Schwartz, "In Vitro Effect of Reiki Treatment on Bacterial Cultures: Role of Experimental Context and Practitioner Well-being," *Journal of Alternative and Complementary Medicine*, no. 12 (2006): 7–13, https://www.ncbi.nlm.nih.gov/pubmed/16494563.

30. Rubik, Brooks, and Schwartz, "In Vitro Effect of Reiki Treatment," 7–13.

31. "Heart Rate Variability," HeartMath Institute, October 27, 2014, https://www.heartmath.org/articles-of-the-heart/the-math-of-heart math/heart-rate-variability/.

32. Fred Shaffer, Rollin McCraty, and Christopher L. Zerr, "A Healthy Heart Is Not a Metronome: An Integrative Review of the Heart's Anatomy and Heart Rate Variability," *Frontiers in Psychology*, no. 5 (2014): 1040.

33. Shaffer, McCraty, and Zerr, "A Healthy Heart," 1040.

34. "HeartMath Purpose and Vision: To Help Activate the Heart of Humanity," HeartMath Institute, https://www.heartmath.com/about/.

35. "Science of the Heart: Exploring the Role of the Heart in Human Performance," HeartMath Institute, https://www.heartmath.org/research/science-of-the-heart/energetic-communication/.

36. "Science of the Heart," HeartMath Institute.

37. Bessel van der Kolk, M.D., "The Importance of Heart Rate Variability on Our Emotional Health and Well-Being," https://www.heartmath.com/blog/articles/hrv-emotional-health-well-being-vanderkolk/.

38. Jay P. Ginsberg, Ph.D., Melanie E. Berry, MS, and Donald A. Powell, Ph.D., "Cardiac Coherence and Posttraumatic Stress Disorder in Combat Veterans," *Alternative Therapies in Health and Medicine*, no. 16 (2010): 52–60, https://www.heartmath.org/assets/uploads/2015/01/cardiac-coherence-and-ptsd-in-combat-veterans.pdf.

39. M. Trousselard et al., "Cardiac Coherence Training to Reduce Anxiety in Remitted Schizophrenia, A Pilot Study," *Applied Psychology and Biofeedback*, no. 41 (2016): 61–69, doi: 10.1007/s10484-015-9312-y.

40. Sonya Kim, Ph.D., CRC, et al., "Heart Rate Variability Biofeedback, Self-Regulation, and Severe Brain Injury," *Biofeedback*, no. 43 (2015): 6–14, doi: 10.5298/1081–5937–43.1.10.

41. "Assimilation and Jean Piaget: Definition, Theory & Process," Study.com, https://study.com/academy/lesson/assimilation-and-piaget-definition -theory-process.html.

42. David J. Hufford, Ph.D., et al., "Barriers to the Entry of Biofield Healing into 'Mainstream' Healthcare," *Biofield Science and Healing: Toward a Transdisciplinary Approach*, no. 4 (2015): 79–88.

43. Hufford et al., "Barriers to the Entry of Biofield Healing," 79–88.

44. Ibid.

CHAPTER 5: THE CHAKRAS

1. Joe Flint, "NBC Bet $69 Million on Megyn Kelly—Then Viewers Vanished," *Wall Street Journal*, April 25, 2018, https://www.wsj.com /articles/nbc-bet-69-million-on-megyn-kellythen-viewers-vanished -1524667220.

2. "Chakra," *New World Encyclopedia*, https://www.newworldencyclo pedia.org/entry/Chakra.

3. Rachel Jacoby Zoldan, "Your 7 Chakras, Explained—Plus How to Tell if They're Blocked," *Well + Good*, August 2, 2018, https://www .wellandgood.com/good-advice/what-are-chakras/.

4. Ben Weiss, "Fractals: A World in a Grain of Sand," filmed for TEDx-VeniceBeach, and published July 24, 2018, https://www.youtube.com /watch?v=DHNooAe44dY.

5. Kate Dektar, "Fractals, Part 3," https://cs.stanford.edu/people/eroberts /courses/soco/projects/2008–09/modeling-natural-systems/fractals3 .html.

6. "What Is the Sacral Chakra?" Chakras.info, http://www.chakras.info /sacral-chakra/.

7. "Gut-Brain Axis," Wikipedia, https://en.wikipedia.org/wiki/Gut%E2 %80%93brain_axis.

8. Leonard A. Wisneski and Lucy Anderson, "The Scientific Basis of Integrative Medicine," *Evidence-based Complementary and Alternative Medicine* vol. 2,2 (2005): 257–59.

9. "Sushumna," Yogapedia, https://www.yogapedia.com/definition/5596 /sushumna.

10. Manoj K. Bhasin et al., "Relaxation Response Induces Temporal

Transcriptome Changes in Energy Metabolism, Insulin Secretion and Inflammatory Pathways," *PLOS One* 8, no. 5 (2013), https://doi.org /10.1371/journal.pone.0062817.

11. Bhasin et al., "Relaxation Response."

12. Masahiro Kumeta et al. "Cell Type-Specific Suppression of Mechano-sensitive Genes by Audible Sound Stimulation," *PLOS One* 13, no. 1 (2018).

13. Hari Sharma, "Ayurveda: Science of Life, Genetics, and Epigenetics." *Ayu* 37, no. 2 (2016): 87–91.

14. Preetha Anand et al., "Cancer Is a Preventable Disease that Requires Major Lifestyle Changes." *Pharmaceutical Research* 25, no. 9 (2008): 2097–116.

15. Hind Sbihi et al., "Perinatal Air Pollution Exposure and Development of Asthma from Birth to Age 10 Years," *European Respiratory Journal* 47, no. 4 (2016): 1062–71.

16. Bailey Kirkpatrick, "Pregnant Moms' Exposure to Pollution May Epigenetically Increase Child's Asthma Susceptibility," Whatisepigenetics .com, August 22, 2017, https://www.whatisepigenetics.com/pregnant -moms-exposure-pollution-may-epigenetically-increase-childs-asthma -susceptibility/.

17. N. P. Kellermann, "Epigenetic Transmission of Holocaust Trauma: Can Nightmares Be Inherited?" *Israel Journal of Psychiatry and Related Sciences* 50, no. 1 (2013): 33–39.

CHAPTER 6: AYURVEDIC MEDICINE

1. Preetha Anand, "Cancer Is a Preventable Disease," 2097–116.

2. Marc A. Shampo, PhD, et al., "J. Craig Venter—The Human Genome Response," *Mayo Clinic Proceedings*, no. 86 (2011).

3. Craig Venter, "DNA of the Future," *India Today*, March 20, 2008, https://www.indiatoday.in/conclave/day-3-march-15–08/story /the-dna-of-the-future-840504–2008–03–15.

4. Christine Kinealy, *This Great Calamity: The Irish Famine, 1845–52* (Dublin: Gill & Macmillan, 1994).

5. Henri A. van der Zee, *The Hunger Winter: Occupied Holland 1944–1945* (Lincoln: University of Nebraska Press, 1998), 304–5.

6. Siddhartha Mukherjee, "Same but Different," *New Yorker*, April 25, 2016, https://www.newyorker.com/magazine/2016/05/02/breakthroughs -in-epigenetics.

7. Carl Zimmer, "The Famine Ended 70 Years Ago, but Dutch Genes Still Bear Scars," *New York Times*, January 31, 2018, https://www.nytimes .com/2018/01/31/science/dutch-famine-genes.html.

8. L. H. Lumey and A. D. Stein, "Transgenerational Effects of Prenatal Exposure to the Dutch Famine," *BJOG: An International Journal of Obstetrics & Gynaecology* 116, no. 6. (May 2009): 868, https://doi.org /10.1111/j.1471–0528.2009.02110.x.

9. Gyan Rajhans, "Pitri-Paksha—Annual Ancestral Worship," Learn Religions, October 1, 2018, https://www.learnreligions.com/pitri-paksha -annual-ancestor-worship-1770146.

10. James Lochtefeld, *The Illustrated Encyclopedia of Hinduism* (New York: Rosen Publishing Group, 2001), 529–30.

11. Sharma, "Ayurveda," 87–91.

CHAPTER 7: THE YOGA OF SOUND

1. "History of Yoga," Yogabasics.com, http://www.yogabasics.com/learn /history-of-yoga/.

2. Karel Werner, *A Popular Dictionary of Hinduism* (London: Curzon Press, 1994).

3. Wendy Doniger, *Textual Sources for the Study of Hinduism*, 1st ed. (Chicago: University of Chicago Press, 1990), 2–3.

4. Robert A. McDermott, "Indian Spirituality in the West: A Bibliographical Mapping," *Philosophy East and West* 25, no. 2 (April 1975): 228–30.

5. Stan van Hooft, ed., *The Handbook of Virtue Ethics* (London and New York: Routledge Taylor & Francis Group, 2014), 302.

6. "Raja Yoga," *New World Encyclopedia*, https://www.newworldencyclo pedia.org/entry/Raja_yoga.

7. W. Y. Evans-Wentz, *Tibetan Yoga and Secret Doctrines*, 3rd ed. (New York: Oxford University Press, 2000), chapters 7 and 8.

8. V. Raghavan et al., *New Catalogus Catalogorum*, 11th ed. (Madras: University of Madras, 1968), 89–90. Lists ten separate authors by the name Patañjali.

9. Dominik Wujastyk, "The Path to Liberation through Yogic Mindfulness in Early Ayurveda," in David Gordon White, ed., *Yoga in Practice* (Princeton, NJ: Princeton University Press, 2011).

10. Elizabeth De Michelis, *A History of Modern Yoga* (New York: Continuum Publishing, 2005).

11. Line Goguen-Huges, "Yoga's Twisted History," *mindful*, February 11, 2011, https://www.mindful.org/yogas-twisted-history/.

12. "When Freud Met Jung," All Psychology Schools, https://www.all psychologyschools.com/psychology/freud-jung/.

13. Anthony Stevens, "The Archetypes," chapter 3 in Renos Papadopoulos, *The Handbook of Jungian Psychology* (New York: Routledge, 2006).

14. James S. Baumlin, Tita French Baumlin, and George H. Jensen, eds., *Post-Jungian Criticism: Theory and Practice* (Albany, NY: SUNY Press, 2004), 192.

15. C. G. Jung, *Aion: Researches into the Phenomenology of the Self* (Collected Works of C. G. Jung, Vol. 9, Part 2) (Princeton, NJ: Princeton University Press; 2nd ed., 1979), 8–11.

16. Marie-Louise von Franz, "The Process of Individuation," in Carl Jung, ed., *Man and His Symbols* (London: Dell Publishing, 1964), 161.

17. "Carl Jung and the Shadow: The Hidden Power of Our Dark Side," Academy of Ideas, https://academyofideas.com/2015/12/carl-jung -and-the-shadow-the-hidden-power-of-our-dark-side/.

18. C. G. Jung, in *Selected Letters of C.G. Jung, 1909–1961*, eds. Gerhard Adler and Aniela Jaffé (Princeton, NJ: Princeton University Press, 1984), 18–19.

19. Jung, *Aion*, 8–11.

20. Robert Aziz, *C. G. Jung's Psychology of Religion and Synchronicity*, 10th ed. (Albany, NY: SUNY Press, 1990).

21. Sannyasi Krishnadhyanam, "Research on Yoga; Nada Yoga: Science of Sound," *YOGA, Magazine of the Bihar School of Yoga*, http://www .yogamag.net/archives/2011/emay11/sound.shtml.

22. Robert J. Zatorre and Valorie N. Salimpoor, "Why Music Makes Our Brain Sing," *New York Times*, June 7, 2013, https://www.nytimes.com /2013/06/09/opinion/sunday/why-music-makes-our-brain-sing.html.

CHAPTER 8: MANTRA

1. G. Feuerstein, *The Deeper Dimension of Yoga* (Boston: Shambhala Publications, 2003).

2. Sakthi Amma, lecture on yoga, at her home Sri Bhavan in Tamil Nadu, India.

3. David Frawley, *Mantra Yoga and the Primal Sound: Secrets of Seed (Bija) Mantras* (Twin Lakes, WI: Lotus Press, 2010), 25.

4. Frawley, *Mantra Yoga*, 31.

5. David Osborn, editor, *Science of the Sacred: Ancient Perspectives for Modern Science* (Lulu.com, 2010).

6. "The Heart Chakra," Chakras.info, https://www.chakras.info/heart -chakra/.

7. Michelle Fondin, "Open Yourself to Love with the Fourth Chakra," Chopra Center, https://chopra.com/articles/open-yourself-to-love-with -the-fourth-chakra?_ga=2.236244802.290485333.1558782549 –1832464967.1558782549.

8. C. G. Jung, *The Red Book: Liber Novus*, tr. M. Kyburz, J. Peck, and S. Shamdasani (New York: W. W. Norton, 2009).

9. Sara Corbett, "The Holy Grail of the Unconscious," *New York Times*, September 6, 2009, https://www.nytimes.com/2009/09/20/magazine /20jung-t.html.

10. C. G. Jung, *The Red Book: Liber Novus*.

11. "About Deva Premal and Miten Band," https://devapremalmiten.com /temple/lyrics-chords/band/.

12. "Cher Gayatri Mantra," published December 5, 2013, https://www .youtube.com/watch?v=WEPBYb1pw8Q.

13. K. T. Weidmann, "Maharishi Mahesh Yogi," in Christian von Dehsen, ed., *Philosophers and Religious Leaders: An Encyclopedia of People Who Changed the World* (Westport, CT: Greenwood, 1999), 120.

14. Philip Goldberg, *American Veda: From Emerson and the Beatles to Yoga and Meditation—How Indian Spirituality Changed the West* (New York: Harmony Books, 2010).

15. "David Lynch Foundation," https://www.davidlynchfoundation.org/.

16. Kate Devlin, "Transcendental Meditation 'Can Treat Depression,'" *Telegraph*, April 7, 2010, https://www.telegraph.co.uk/news/health /news/7563648/Transcendental-meditation-can-treat-depression .html.

17. Ron Jevning, "Adrenocortical Activity during Meditation," *Hormones and Behavior* 10, no. 1 (1978): 54–60.

18. Kenneth R. Eppley, Allan I. Abrams, and Jonathan Shear, "Differential Effects of Relaxation Techniques on Trait Anxiety: A Meta-Analysis," *Journal of Clinical Psychology* 45, no. 6 (1989): 957–74.

19. Maharishi University of Management, "$2.4 Million Grant to Study the Transcendental Meditation Program and PTSD in Veterans," December 2, 2012, www.mum.edu/Customized/uploads/publications /achievements/2012_12_02.html.

20. Sarina J. Grosswald et al., "Use of the Transcendental Meditation Technique to Reduce Symptoms of Attention Deficit Hyperactivity Disorder (ADHD) by Reducing Stress and Anxiety: An Exploratory Study," *Current Issues in Education*, 10 (2008), https://cie.asu.edu/ojs /index.php/cieatasu/article/view/1569.

21. Jennie Rothenberg Gritz, "Mantras Before Math Class," *Atlantic*, November 10, 2015, https://www.theatlantic.com/education/archive /2015/11/mantras-before-math-class/412618/.

22. "Quiet Time Changes Lives," David Lynch Foundation, https://www .davidlynchfoundation.org/schools.html.

23. Robert H. Schneider et al., "Stress Reduction in the Secondary Prevention of Cardiovascular Disease," *Circulation: Cardiovascular Quality and Outcomes* 5, no. 6 (2012): 750–58, https://doi.org /10.1161/circoutcomes.112.967406.

24. "Meditation and Cardiovascular Risk Reduction: A Scientific Statement from the American Heart Association," *Journal of the American Heart Association* 6, no. 10 (2017), https://doi.org/10.1161/JAHA.117.002218.

25. "Tour of the Electromagnetic Spectrum," NASA Science, https://sci ence.nasa.gov/ems/02_anatomy?fbclid=IwAR1AV9XQMAvaSiCE mJw0lp_u_DmtZHif8HcbA_vwWN_0qYM3xPsVbWgYnVI.

26. Igor Jerman, Robert Leskovar, and R. Krašovec, "Evidence for Biofield," in *Philosophical Insights about Modern Science*, ed. Eva Zerovnik, Olga Markič, and Andrej Ule (Hauppauge, NY: Nova Science Publishers, 2009), 199–216.

27. John Hubacher, "The Phantom Leaf Effect: A Replication, Part 1," *Journal of Alternative and Complementary Medicine* 21, no. 2 (2015), https://doi.org/10.1089/acm.2013.0182.

28. Jiří Pokorný et al, "Electromagnetic Field of Microtubules: Effects on Transfer of Mass Particles and Electrons," *Journal of Biological Physics* 31, no. 3–4 (2005): 501–14, doi: 10.1007/s10867-005-1286-1.

29. David Muehsam and Carlo Ventura, "Life Rhythm as a Symphony of Oscillatory Patterns: Electromagnetic Energy and Sound Vibration Modulates Gene Expression for Biological Signaling and Healing," *Global Advances in Health and Medicine* 3, no. 2 (2014): 40–55, doi: 10.7453/gahmj.2014.008.

30. Muehsam and Ventura, "Life Rhythm," 40–55.

31. Roy K. Aaron and Deborah Mck. Ciombor, "Therapeutic Effects of Electromagnetic Fields in the Stimulation of Connective Tissue

Repair," *Journal of Cellular Biochemistry* 52, no. 1 (1993): 42–46. https://doi.org/10.1002/jcb.240520107.

32. "Electric Cures," *Scientific American*, 312, no. 3 (March 2015).

33. Beverly Rubik, "Sympathetic Resonance Technology™: Scientific Foundation and Summary of Biologic and Clinical Studies," *Journal of Alternative and Complementary Medicine* 8, no. 6 (2002): 823–56, https://doi.org/10.1089/10755530260511838.

34. James K. Gimzewski, Andrew E. Pelling, and Carlo Ventura, international patent for "Nanomechanical Characterization of Cellular Activity," September 4, 2008, International Publication Number WO 2008/105919 A2, https://patents.google.com/patent/WO2008105919A2/en.

35. Beverly Rubik, Ph.D., "Measurement of the Human Biofield and Other Energetic Instruments/Chapter 20 of 'Energetics and Spirituality' by Lyn Freeman," Foundation for Alternative and Integrative Medicine, https://www.faim.org/measurement-of-the-human-biofield-and-other-energetic-instruments.

CHAPTER 9: THE SIDDHAS

1. Sanchita Sharma, "Dravidian Language Family Is 4,500 Years Old, Finds International Study," *Hindustan Times*, March 21, 2018, https://www.hindustantimes.com/india-news/dravidian-language-family-is-4–500-years-old-finds-international-study/story-xRsAAzj5wqOIVPAgd3TkWL.html.

2. K. S. Uthamarayan, *Siddha Maruthuvanga Surukkam* (Chennai, India: Department of Indian Medicine and Homoeopathy, third edition, 2003).

3. K. V. Ramakrishna Rao, "A Critical Study of the Chronology of Siddhas," Hinduwebsite.com, https://www.hinduwebsite.com/hinduism/essays/siddhas.asp.

4. Rao, "A Critical Study of the Chronology of Siddhas."

5. Stuart Alve Olson, *Qigong Teachings of a Taoist Immortal: The Eight Essential Exercises of Master Li Ching-Yun* (Rochester, VT: Bear & Company, 2002).

6. M. Krishnaveni et al., "Siddhar's Methods of Processing Therapeutic Mercury," https://www.researchgate.net/publication/36447893_Siddhar's_methods_of_processing_therapeutic_Mercury.

7. "Tapas/Hinduism," *Encyclopedia Britannica*, https://www.britannica.com/topic/tapas.

8. Swami Ayyappa Giri and Yogini Ashram, "Forests, Mountains, Temples, and Caves of Agastya," January 16, 2018, https://www.yoginiashram.com/siddha-agastya-lopamudrai-kriya-babaji/.

9. Palpandian, *Siddhas: Masters of the Basics*, 2nd ed. (Chennai: Achala Siddha, 2008).

10. Palpandian, *Siddhas*.

11. Palpandian, *Siddhas*.

12. Jane Bosveld, "Isaac Newton, World's Most Famous Alchemist," *Discover*, December 28, 2010, http://discovermagazine.com/2010/jul-aug/05-isaac-newton-worlds-most-famous-alchemist.

13. Andrea Pflaumer, "Kaya Kalpa: Life Extension and Immortality," Michael Laughrin's North American Jyotish Newsletter, June/July 2009, http://jyotish.ws/wisdom/kaya_kalpa_immortality.html.

14. Pflaumer, "Kaya Kalpa."

15. Nirmal Sengupta, *Economic Studies of Indigenous and Traditional Knowledge* (New Delhi: Academic Foundation and the Indian Economic Association Trust, 2007).

16. Barun Kumar De, *Public System Management* (New Delhi: New Age International Publishers, 2006).

17. Ministry of AYUSH, http://ayush.gov.in/.

18. Richard S. Weiss, *Recipes for Immortality: Healing, Religion, and Community in South India* (New York: Oxford University Press, 2009), 93.

19. Surendra Pathak, M.D., "Harmony Exists Universally from Microcosm to Macrocosm: Peaceful Coexistence Is the Nature of Everything" (Conference paper, 2014), https://www.researchgate.net/publication/269897711_Harmony_exists_universally_from_Microcosm_to_Macrocosm_Peaceful_Coexistence_is_the_Nature_of_everything.

20. Menas C. Kafatos et al., "Biofield Science: Current Physics Perspectives," *Global Advances in Health and Medicine* 4, Suppl. (2015): 25–34, doi: 10.7453/gahmj.2015.011.suppl.

INDEX